# Spirituality *in* Nursing
## 2nd Edition
### From Traditional to New Age

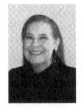

**Barbara Stevens Barnum, RN, PhD, FAAN,** consultant and author, is a former editor of *Nursing Leadership Forum.* In her career, she held appointments as editor of *Nursing & Health Care,* and served in positions at both Columbia University programs of nursing, including holding the directorship, Division of Health Services, Sciences, and Education at Teachers College, where she also held the Stewart Chair and chairmanship in the Department of Nursing Education. Dr. Barnum is presently an adjunct professor at the Columbia University School of Nursing.

In Chicago, Dr. Barnum coordinated the Nursing Service Administration Program of the College of Nursing, University of Illinois, and held administrative posts at the University of Chicago Hospitals and at Augustana Hospital and Health Care Center.

Dr. Barnum has written widely in areas of nursing management, theory, education, and aspects of spirituality/holistic nursing. Her books include: *Nursing Theory: Analysis, Application, Evaluation* (6th ed. underway); *The Nurse as Executive* (4th ed.), (with K. Kerfoot); *Writing for Publication: A Primer for Nurses*; and *The New Healer: Minds and Hands in Complementary Medicine.*

A fellow of the American Academy of Nursing, Dr. Barnum has done extensive national and international consultation and continuing education, including an eight-year term as consultant to the Air Force Surgeon General. Dr. Barnum presently conducts workshops in areas of complementary medicine and spirituality. She has two books underway: one on mysticism and the other on the psychopharmacology of psychiatry (with E. DiFrancesco). Dr. Barnum also writes fiction—*The Haunting of Lila Tilden* is her first published novel.

# Spirituality *in* Nursing
## 2nd Edition
### From Traditional to New Age

Barbara Stevens Barnum, RN, PhD, FAAN

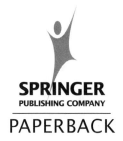

**SPRINGER**
PUBLISHING COMPANY

PAPERBACK

Springer Publishing Company, Inc.
11 West 42nd Street
New York, NY 10036

Acquisitions Editor: Ruth Chasek
Production Editor: Jeanne W. Libby
Cover design by Mimi Flow

06  07  08  09  /  5  4  3  2  1

New ISBN 0-8261-9182-7 © 2006 by Springer Publishing Company, Inc.

---

**Library of Congress Cataloging-in-Publication Data**

Barnum, Barbara Stevens.
    Spirituality in nursing : from traditional to new age / Barbara
Stevens Barnurn.—2nd ed.
        p. ; cm.
    includes bibliographical references and index.
    ISBN 0-8261-9181-9
    1. Nursing—Religious aspects. 2. Nursing—Philosophy.
  3. Nursing—Psychological aspects. 4. Spirituality. I. Title.
    [DNLM: 1. Philosophy, Nursing. 2. Religion and Medicine.
  3. Spirituality. WY 86 B263s 2003]
RT85.2.B37 2003
610.73'01—dc21                                 2003042361

---

Printed in the United States of America by Bang Printing.

## Dedication

This book is dedicated to my daughter, Lauren Stevens, who designed the cover for this and the previous edition. I'm very fortunate to have Lauren as a daughter, and doubly blessed that she has a career as an Art Director. Much of her artistry has been spent in designing book covers and advertisements for books, so I take advantage of her expertise. It may be superstitious, but I'm convinced that my books do better when she designs the covers.

Thank you, Lauren, for never complaining when I ask for yet another cover—at a mother's "price," namely *gratis* except for dinners out.

# Contents

*Preface to the Second Edition*                                          ix

**Part I   Spirituality Today and Yesterday**
  1   Spirituality in Nursing: Past and Present Trends                    5
  2   Spirituality and Nursing's History                                 21

**Part II   Spirituality and the Emerging Paradigm**
  3   Spirituality, Physics, Philosophy, and Psychology                  37
  4   Developmental Theories: Is There a Spiritual Phase?                51

**Part III   Spirituality and the Individual**
  5   Spirituality and the Mind                                          71
  6   Spirituality and the Brain                                         79
  7   Spirituality, Illness, and Death                                   93

**Part IV   Spirituality in Nursing's New Paradigm**
  8   Spirituality as a Component in Nursing Theories                   107
  9   Nursing Theorists in the New Paradigm                             113
 10   Nursing and Healing                                               129

**Part V   Spiritual Interventions in Health Care**
 11   Spiritual and New Age Therapeutics                                141
 12   Spirituality, Traditional Religion, and Traditional
      Therapeutics                                                      163

**Part VI   Spirituality and Ethics**
 13   Spirituality and Ethics: A Contrast in Forms                      185
 14   Ethics and Philosophy                                             195

*Index*                                                                 201

# Preface to the Second Edition

When the first edition of this book was written, spirituality was just reentering nursing's interest and practice. In the interim time, nursing's focus on spirituality has only grown. Yet attention to spirituality by the profession has waxed and waned over the decades. Indeed, nursing as a discrete profession arose from spirituality, then relegated spirituality to a back seat in its drive to become credible in the academic world. Now nursing is turning back to see what was lost in this maneuver.

This book looks at nursing's relationship with spirituality from various perspectives: theoretical, historical, religious, psychological, and physiological. It examines the renewed interest in spirituality fostered by the so-called New Age Movement in the larger society. The book reviews spirituality as a nursing task and asks, are we prepared to tackle it? It considers spirituality as a patient need and as a nursing diagnosis. It weighs spirituality as a nursing domain in competition with the spiritual ministration rights claimed by chaplains, other religious practitioners, and physicians who have recently jumped on the "spiritual bandwagon." It ponders the nature of spirituality reflected in our newer and older nursing theories. It compares and contrasts spiritual remedies offered in traditional and New Age philosophies.

The book is not meant to be a compendium on the subject matter of spirituality. Instead, it is an intimate look at the thoughts of one nurse on spirituality as it affects our work in a profession that puts us in intimate interaction with other human beings at stressful and meaningful times in their lives.

However one views spirit and spirituality, the quest for ultimate meaning in life rears its head in the practice of nursing in at least three guises. First, nurses must be concerned with their own concepts of spirit, their own ways of giving meaning to their lives. Second, they must confront patients in moments of stress that bring to the forefront the patients' spiritual concerns. Third, nurses must consider how ethics and spirituality inform the organizations in which they work.

# PART I

## Spirituality Today and Yesterday

*Spirituality* is a term frequently heard in nursing as well as in the society at large. Yet the term means different things to different people. At one extreme, it appears to be a catchword for anything with a humanitarian bent. At the other extreme, spirituality is closely associated with one's specific religion. For purposes of this book, the term *spirituality* will mean a person's search for, or expression of, his connection to a greater and meaningful context. For some people, that will be seen as a connection with God; for others it may be finding their place in the universe, and that may involve in-depth searching for a greater sense of self. On a metaphysical level, spirituality can involve asking, "Who am I?"

For some the search is religious, for others philosophical, and yet for others humanitarian. Spirituality creates an urge to locate oneself in the greater circle of meaning, to understand one's existence, and to reflect on one's place in the cosmos.

Although the spiritual may be accessed by learning, its tone is not scholarly. The modifiers that come to mind in thinking of spirit are words like *awe, inspiration*, and *reverence*. These elements make clear that spirituality is more than merely a humanitarian motive.

As Lama Surya Das (1999) describes it:

Whatever words we choose to use, spiritual matters concern themselves with the true bottom line, with those things that really matter in the long run. As spiritual seekers, we think about how we can learn to love more deeply, know ourselves more truly, and connect with the divine more fully.

We think about those things that are beyond the self; we think about the intangible; we think about the visible and the invisible; we think about touching the palpable sweetness of spirit; we think about how we can find ourselves in the whole, the bigger picture, the universal "mandala." (pp. 9–10)

Burkhardt and Jacobson (2000) elaborate on these same elements:

Spirituality permeates life; shapes our life journey; and is vital to the process of discovering purpose, meaning, and inner strength. (p. 94)

Dossey and Guzzetta (2000) say that spirit is

[a] unifying force of a person; the essence of being that permeates all of life and is manifested in one's being, knowing, and doing; the interconnectedness with self, others, nature, and God/Life Force/Absolute/ Transcendent. (p. 7)

These descriptions capture the sense of spirituality used throughout this book. Notice that both Lama Surya Das and all the nurse authors express the context in which one lives rather than specific content. Hence, spirituality may be reflected in humanitarian acts, in religion, or in many different ways. Alternately it is possible to have both humanitarian acts and religious practices that stem from nonspiritual motives. Spirituality, then, is a context and a motive, a search, and, for many, a search successfully concluded.

Part I reviews spirituality in nursing, starting with today and moving backward through time. Chapter 1 orients the reader to the trends that gave rise to today's resurgence of interest in spirituality. Why are matters of the spirit suddenly of concern to nurses everywhere? Chapter 1 proposes three major reasons.

Chapter 2 looks at selected aspects of nursing's spiritual history and origins. The assets and limitations of nursing in the past are considered. For example, in the Dark Ages and before, a little religious comfort—a prayer, a reading from the Bible—was the most that a nurse could offer a patient. Why in today's era of high technology is the nurse returning to forms of spiritual ministration? How many nurses remember the Greek goddesses associated with early nursing? How many nurses know that Nightingale wrote meditations and even began a serious book on fourteenth century Christian mystics?

Our historical roots are complex and interesting and add a dimension to nursing that brings us a depth of understanding of our spiritual heritage.

## REFERENCES

Burkhardt, M. A., & Jacobson, M. G. N. (2000). Spirituality and health. In B. M. Dossey, L. Keegan, & C. E. Guzzetta (Eds.), *Holistic nursing: A handbook for practice* (3rd ed., pp. 91–122). Gaithersburg, MD: Aspen.

Dossey, B. M., & Guzzetta, C. E. (2000). Holistic nursing practice. In B. M. Dossey, L. Keegan, & C. E. Guzzetta (Eds.), *Holistic nursing: A handbook for practice* (3rd ed., pp. 5–33). Gaithersburg, MD: Aspen.

Lama Surya Das (1999). *Awakening to the sacred.* New York: Random House.

# Chapter 1

## Spirituality in Nursing: Past and Present Trends

In the last decade, spirituality has burst back on the scene in nursing. At least three forces are at work in the renewed focus: (1) a major shift in the normative world view, that is, the prevailing social paradigm by which reality is interpreted; (2) a spiritual focus in the growing self-help movement; and (3) a renewed attention to the spiritual impact (intended or incidental) of implementing new care delivery models. Of these, the shift in the world view is the major factor.

### THE NEW VERSUS THE OLD PARADIGM: A CHANGING WORLD VIEW

It is common for the professions, including nursing, to follow trends in the larger society, and our profession has been in the midst of change for more than two decades. Even those who do not admit to a *major* paradigm shift recognize a new and growing minority who point out the limitations of the scientific world model. Whether major paradigm shift or a minority position, the new perspective attempts to flesh out the scientific interpretation from a larger perspective, one with room for experiences and phenomena long denied under the rationalistic rules.

One aspect of human reality that is given credence under the new paradigm is man's eternal search for the meaning of his existence and the meaning of reality. In other words, spirituality arises as a valid domain in the new paradigm. Society's renewed interest in spirituality is evident in everything from television to workshops to popular magazines. Books concerning spirituality that once would have had a small audience have become best sellers. Moore (1994), Hillman (1996), Peck (1997), and Zukav (1989) revitalized the term *soul*. They advocate something both old and new: that man bring

5

spirituality into his everyday life, that he recognize the existence of his soul apart from his body and its neurochemistry. New syntheses are taking place under the emerging paradigm, with Zukav (2001) showing how physics and mysticism reveal surprisingly similar patterns, and Myss (1996) interweaving Eastern notions of the chakra system with the ideas in the Christian and Jewish sacraments.

To these infusions of spirituality are added Eastern influences. Kabat-Zinn (1994) and numerous books by the Dalai Lama, such as *The Art of Happiness* (with Cutler, 1998), illustrate this trend. These and similar books introduce principles of Buddhism or Zen Buddhism with their practices such as living in the moment and meditation.

These practices arising in the new paradigm have been adopted extensively by the larger society. If these fermenting ideas related to spirituality (traditional, New Age, Eastern) have not created a new social paradigm, they have certainly created a broadly practiced counterculture. It is not surprising that such practices infiltrated from the broader society into traditional medicine.

### Paradigm Shift in General Health Care

We've already seen radical changes in perception among medics concerning alternative medicine practices associated with Eastern spiritual traditions. One finds meditation, for example, advocated in such conditions as stress and hypertension. One even finds employee meditation groups gathering over lunch hours in many businesses. One also finds patients and staff on inpatient units following the same procedure.

Research on complementary medicine has moved from its first federal recognition in the Office of Alternative Medicine to a larger presence in the National Center for Complementary and Alternative Medicine Research in the National Institutes of Health. Hence, testing of many practices emerging from spiritual philosophies have been legitimated.

Among complementary health care practices, many methods are associated with altered states of consciousness on the part of the practitioner, like energy movement systems (e.g., Reiki or therapeutic touch). Others involve altered states on the part of the patient, like meditation and biofeedback. Many forms of spirituality also involve altered states of mind, ranging from newer forms of religious contemplation to Buddhist meditation. In other words, there is a renewed interest in forms of spirituality and forms of therapy associated with altered states of mind.

As the new paradigm infiltrated health care, early adjustments were often pragmatic. Therapies that did not fit the old scientific world-view were adopted despite resistance. If acupuncture worked, it was no longer discarded just because it *should not* work according to the medical theory of cell, organ, system, integrated systems. Acupuncture, based on an entirely different and Eastern philosophy of man, began to appear in credible research in major institutions— for example Anastasi's (Anastasi, Dawes, & Ming, 1997; Barnum, 2002) research on acupuncture to control diarrhea in HIV patients. And if past life therapy cured major neurotic patterns, psychiatrists and psychologists decided it didn't matter whether the past lives were real or not. If the therapy worked, it was used.

Of course, effective new therapies arising out of a changed paradigm encourage changing one's beliefs to be consistent with the therapies. If the therapy precedes the philosophy, it serves as a stimulus for new thought. For example, if a health practitioner sees that Reiki energy movement works, he begins to search for a world-view to explain this finding. In turn, changes in the world-view cause people to seek out therapies congruent with the changing model. Numerous new practitioners have appeared on the health scene, including Rolfers, cranio-sacral therapists, reflexologists, sound therapists, essential oils and aroma therapists, Reiki practitioners, thought-field therapists, and past lives therapists to name but a few (Barnum, 2002). And these practitioners bring with them alternate views of reality, often including so-called New Age elements of spirituality.

Among other changes, therapists under the new paradigm perceive and treat the mind in a new way, namely as a tool for healing. Patients are taught imagery to fight cancer, biofeedback to lower blood pressure, and hypnotism to stop smoking. The old image of psychosomatic disease has changed. Instead of *psychosomatic* being a term for the body *fooling* itself, the phenomenon has come to be recognized as a tool for the body to *heal* itself.

The pragmatic appeal of spirituality (even traditional religion) got a major boost in medicine when religious patients were found to have better medical outcomes. Of course there is an irony in treating spirituality and religion as mere tools for improved medical outcomes, but that happens frequently. Physician Matthews (1997) illustrates this perspectives.

> Religious practices and beliefs, for the most part appear to be good for one's health. The medical effect of prayer and healing seems to be more related to the intensity of one's own practices and belief system, than to the particular denomination or religious tradition with which one is affiliated. Based on limited data, devout people of various religions appear to have similar medical effects. (p. 18)

Although it seems hypocritical, it is not surprising that spirituality is seen as a means of serving the ends of medicine. This is not to say that the conditions of illness have not often served as a stimulus toward a renewed search for spirituality.

Nowhere is the conflict between the new and the older paradigm better illustrated than in the work of Prince and Reiss (1990). They struggle in the practice of psychiatry against the constraints of the scientific world-view, noting that the selected explanatory model has impact on the care patients subsequently receive. For example, Prince and Reiss note that the labeling of persons as psychotic immediately alters their care. From a different paradigm, some of these persons might be seen as normal. In many cultures, for example, the hallucinations of shamans are seen as sacred psychological states.

Prince and Reiss extend their perspective beyond shamanism to those labeled more frankly psychotic:

> In the Western world, when psychotics speak of their subjective experiences and the supernatural beliefs which often arise from them (delusions in psychiatric parlance), they are rejected by their more rationalistic confreres. (p. 138)
>
> The usual reaction of the psychiatrist (but not necessarily of the lay reader) to ideas such as are expressed in this piece is to dismiss them as delusional and psychotic. The psychiatrist will pay little attention to their contents, apart from noting their formal aspects and as having relevance to diagnostic criteria. . . .
>
> In dismissing these ideas as meaningless, the psychiatrist relegates highly significant experiences of the patient to limbo. Concerns that are of most importance to the patient are irrelevant to the psychiatrist. . . . For the psychiatrist, the explanatory model (EM) of the patient with respect to his or her experience is completely unrealistic and even more damaging, non-negotiable. (p. 141)

Prince and Reiss lay bare the issue between paradigms, and the paradigm question has direct impact on the issue of spirituality. The meaning of spirituality is different in different world-views, but for Prince and Reiss the meaning must be found in what has meaning for the patient.

### Changes in Nursing Under the New Paradigm

As a profession, nursing has not been immune to these new paradigm changes. Of course, this was not the first time that nursing has reacted to changing societal paradigms. For example, when hospital schools of nursing arose historically, students of nursing in this country were taught to care for the body, mind, and spirit of the patient. Nursing literature in the '30s and '40s assumed and applied this model. The prescriptions for care of the spirit may have been limited, but they existed. For example, it was valid nursing work to read the Bible to a patient or to pray with him.

When nursing matured as an aspiring profession, however, it adopted the Western world paradigm, one that featured a scientific viewpoint asserting that everything "real" could be subjected to scientific inquiry. All else was discounted as illusory. Belief in God was interpreted as unsophisticated, belief in a life after death as childish wish fulfillment. Scientists looked down on the uneducated masses who held to such primitive beliefs. As Grof and Grof (1989) asserted:

> The world view created by traditional Western science and dominating our culture is, in its most rigorous form, incompatible with any notion of spirituality. In a universe where only the tangible, material, and measurable are real, all forms of religious and mystical activities are seen as reflecting ignorance, superstition, and irrationality or emotional immaturity. Direct experiences of spiritual realities are then interpreted as "psychotic"—manifestations of mental disease. (p. 3)

Nursing, in its attempt to be contemporary and to model itself after medicine, was quick to follow the new scientific paradigm. Indeed, the conversion to a scientific viewpoint was essential if nursing were to enter the turf of academia, which was its major goal. It was no time to base one's ideology on things that couldn't be measured and subjected to research.

Hence, nurses no longer took care of mind, body, and spirit; instead, they cared for a bio-psycho-social being. True, there were diseases of the body and mind, but no one referred to diseases of the spirit. Fractured bits and pieces of spirituality, if any, were subsumed under aspects of psychology and sociology. As Donley (1991) noted:

> Doctors acted like scientists, businessmen, or entrepreneurs. Nurses were also coopted by the glamour and power of high-technology nursing. As some of the art and most of the mystery of healing were lost, it became clear to nurses, and others who worked in hospitals, that they were part of a technical money-making system, not a "sacred system." (p. 178)

In the education of nurses, required church attendance, popular in religious-affiliated schools up until the early 1950s, was dropped. Attendance at religious ceremonies ceased or was optional. Fewer schools of nursing were associated with religious organizations. Those that were carefully sanitized their curricula.

Spiritual course content was reduced to a sociologic review of the major religions and their applicable tenets. The major religions of this nation were given "equal time" but only in relation to learning special dietary practices and rituals of religious practice that might affect nursing. In this way, spiritual matters became content, not concepts to be considered as value laden. This was quite different from earlier eras when the nurse was infused with a religious or spiritual zeal. True, people still had their beliefs, but those were the territory for chaplains, ministers, priests, or other spiritual leaders. For most intents and purposes, nurses were out of the spirit game.

Indeed, the change from a spiritual to a psychosocial focus was resisted only by the rare school or care delivery institutions. After all, there was so much exciting new information concerning the psychosocial aspects of a patient's being. Psychosomatic disease was a fast growing concept that explained all the necessary linkages. In nursing, as in the larger society, religion and spirituality were taking a back seat to other human ventures and interests.

As long as the scientific, what-you-see-is-what-you-get world-view pertained, nurses and patients alike functioned under the same paradigm. If an occasional nurse found herself in an awkward position because of her personal beliefs, usually the situation could be reconciled.

Then things started to change again. The limitations of the scientific world-view began to pinch. Things kept escaping through the cracks; it became difficult to explain away certain patterns and observations that did not fit the model.

Today in nursing the two world paradigms appear to be conflicting camps. They have yet to reach an adequate synthesis, and there is resistance from each side to the other. Many nurse practitioner programs, for example, are based entirely on the older scientific model. Yet other programs, usually those with some commitment to a holistic philosophy, have a spiritual element and arise from the new paradigm. Therapies in these newer paradigm programs focus on such tactics as therapeutic touch, visualization, and meditation. Unfortunately but not surprisingly, we have few programs that avail themselves of the benefits to be found in both paradigms. Nor is this to say that all holistic nursing is practiced in a spiritual context.

As nursing, or segments of it, moved into the new paradigm, disparate views of spirit emerged. Several of these theories will be contrasted in Chapter 9. One view, typified by Newman (2000), sees mind in the form of expanding consciousness, as what truly comprises man. In this view, expanding consciousness becomes the equivalent of spirit. From another viewpoint, typified by Dossey and Guzzetta (2000), spirit is added as a new component of man that is different from, and not substituted for, the biopsychosocial elements. In other theories, typified by Watson (1999), man is primarily a soul or spirit, and soul does not equate with mind, although body, mind, and soul are inseparable components. Although the latter viewpoint is traditional, it was supplanted for decades and is only now being renewed under the emerging paradigm.

In summary, society, health care, medical care, and nursing have all responded to the new paradigm. This paradigm is evidenced in many different formats. Most of these philosophies are not only compatible with elements of spirit, but in many instances have a spiritual element as foundation.

## THE SPIRITUAL ELEMENT IN SELF-HELP PROGRAMS

One of the few arenas of care where a spiritual component is more common than not is the treatment of alcohol and drug abuse. Typically these programs are multidisciplinary, not invoking the development of unique nursing theories. Most therapy models are based on the philosophy of Alcoholics Anonymous (AA), the first large-scale success in containing substance abuse. Bauer (1982) claims that the AA program succeeded by taking away moral guilt, offering hope, restoring dignity, and respecting one's individuality and the need to remain in the collective society.

The keystone of the AA program was provided by C. G. Jung, who believed that the abuse of alcohol was a defective search for the spiritual. The cure for alcoholism, he said, was to be found in the spirit. Alcohol was the equivalent, on a low level, of spiritual thirst for wholeness; it represented the search for union with God (Bauer, 1982). Jung added:

> You see, "alcohol" in Latin is *spiritus*, and you use the same word for the highest religious experience as well as for the most depraving poison. The helpful formula therefore is: *spiritus contra spiritum*. (Bauer, 1982, p. 127)

The most successful approach in treating substance abuse so far, the 12-step AA program and its clones in drug abuse (for example, Cocaine Anonymous and Narcotics Anonymous), ground recovery in a relationship to a higher power. In regaining this missing sense of spirit, the abuser regains his relationship to a higher power. Although there is no attempt to link these programs to a specific religion, the notion of a higher power is taken quite literally.

AA and its spiritual approach is not new, but the extension of the principle into all domains of the recovery and self-help movement has made it important in returning man's interest to the spiritual. Is substance abuse a natural backlash in a society seriously divorced from spiritual values? Is the rampant substance abuse of this age an ironic, thwarted search for spirit, as Jung believed? A good argument could be made for the case.

Notice the verbal imagery involved. Is drug *intoxication* a poor man's spiritual *intoxication*? Is it coincidence that one *gets high* on drugs just as religions point *heavenward*? Or that many psychedelic users claim they are hooked on another reality revealed by the drug?

Whether or not one agrees that the deficit is spiritual, mere body cure (namely, withdrawal and detoxification) seldom works a cure in substance abusers. Effective rehabilitation programs must offer more than just a substance-free state. As Gold (1984) says in relation to cocaine abuse, one must fill the cocaine hours—the time that was previously filled with thinking about the drug, purchasing it, using it, hanging around with fellow abusers. AA and its imitators fill the abuse hours with a spiritual focus.

Drug abuse today focuses on psychedelics and other intoxicants used in so-called raves, those all-night parties featuring music, drugs, and various psychostimulating experiences. Cox (2002) identifies the most popular drugs as MDMA (Ecstasy), 4-PMA, Nexus (Afterburner), GHB (Liquid X), Ketamine (Special K), and PCP (Angel Dust). Even more than alcohol, these psychedelic drugs illustrate the principle that drugs may be a substitute for more valid spiritual experience. Indeed, the use is reminiscent of the more controlled use of mescaline to produce spiritual visions among Native Americans. George (1995) describes the religious and artistic use of peyote, a small, spineless cactus growing in the Rio Grande Valley and adjacent regions of Mexico and Texas:

> The crowns of the peyote cactus contain the powerful alkaloid hallucinogen mescaline. The ingestion of these crowns, called "mescal buttons" or "peyote buttons," has been one of the most widely used chemical pathways to unusual experiences in native North America. (p. 215)

The self-help movement has grown into arenas once seen to be the domain only of professionals. For example, in psychotherapeutics Santoro and Cohen (1997) offer self help for borderline personality disorders as well as for addictive behaviors. Such an approach not only returns controls to the impaired individual but also, by implication, returns accountability—a notion that is in keeping with a notion of soul and self, as opposed to viewing man as merely a victim of his circumstances.

Self-help (which implies a deficit in some arena of life) has been joined under the new paradigm by a growth in self-improvement programs, even for those seen as well but interested in further self-development. Often such systems are related to New Age notions of spirituality. Weekend conferences and workshops feature everything from rebirthing, to shamanistic vision quests, to breath control (altering the chemical balance of the body), to drumming (auditory driving)—all techniques designed to alter the state of consciousness in those seeking greater knowledge of the inner self or the larger reality. These alterations impact on the themes of spirituality as we have defined it. Sometimes legal or illegal use of psychedelics is involved in such searches for the meaning of self with all the complications that may arise from such use.

Whatever the impetus, the search for self and self-help arise more comfortably under the new paradigm than under the old. Often the self-oriented journeys are tied to one or another interpretation of spirituality. Reintroduction of old shamanic patterns of belief (Barnum, 2002) as well as new interpretations of humans as primarily energy phenomena are included. In nursing, this latter trend can be traced back to Rogers (1970, 1994), although the impetus for these interpretations in our time often comes from recent societal changes.

## SPIRITUAL IMPACT OF IMPLEMENTING NEW CARE DELIVERY MODELS

Health care delivery systems have been going through many reorganizations in recent years. These new care models often affect the environment in ways that foster or stress client and staff spirituality. Some of these effects are deliberate, purposefully creating positive environments that enhance attention to spirituality. In other cases the nature of the new environments tests or frustrates one's capacity for spirituality.

### Intended Effects in New Care Delivery Structures

Systems effects that foster spirituality take place on many levels: (1) adding new practices, (2) modifying the context, that is the environment, or (3) creating new organizing patterns.

#### *Adding New Practices*

Earlier we mentioned the practice of meditation periods for staff and patients. This practice is a good example of a relatively new (in this country and on a large scale) spiritually related practice. Meditation has been instituted on many inpatient units across the nation. Other new practices enhance one's capacity for a spiritual focus by giving more attention to patients as human beings. For example, one might cite the accreditation requirement that pain levels be tracked and relief measures be directed to pain control.

Just as the self-help industry has burgeoned, so has the self-care health industry, with the self-medication growth in herbology chief among the new practices. No industry has grown faster. Similarly, many new health care practitioners of a New Age variety are now available, and many of these relate their practices to a spiritually based philosophy. As Lynne Austin, RN and sound therapist, says (Barnum, 2002):

> Sound is sacred. As our breath is a connection with God, we breathe in the love, light, and energy and exhale through the sounds and tones the perfection of who we are. Sound is also made sacred by the intention behind it. I believe in the beginning of time the intention was love. If we use sound with the intention of love behind it, it brings us into that Christ consciousness and what this master stood for. (p. 32)

Or as Mary Bernau-Eigen, BSN, Rolfer, says (Barnum, 2002) concerning her process when a client is "stuck":

> [t]hen I say to myself, *I need help here.* Or the client might say that he needs help. Then I ask, "What is the healing presence for you?" It might be Jesus, Buddha, Allah, or whoever. Then we bring that presence in. The more we can stick with the client's belief system the better. (p. 85)

New healers and practitioners such as Austin and Bernau-Eigen not only change the health care practices in a spiritually aware direction, but they also change the health care structures and context, creating offices and centers of care where such spirit-sensitive services are available.

### Modifying the Context

Changing the context in which care is given can happen in many ways. As noted above, many new providers gain popularity partially because their services are sensitive to spiritual aspects of the human being. Such attention to environment is happening in traditional institutions as well. St. Luke's Episcopal Hospital in Houston, Texas, for example, gave its environment major scrutiny. On its Healing Environment Committee (St. Luke's, videotape, n.d.), chaplains and other professionals made environmental changes to help patients realize healing.

Actions of the committee included such things as creating nature murals, altering lighting, designing an artificial tree to make an intensive care unit less hostile, creating an effect of clouds in skylights, and providing an internal TV channel with relaxation tapes that feature natural scenes and calming music, to name a few. These changes were perceived as improving ambiance in a religious context.

Such efforts are seen across the nation, improving the patient's environment through attention to the environment. Videotapes like *Rafting Through Canyons at Dawn*, produced by The Environmental Television Network (1995), are available and marketed to health care institutions. Compact disks such as Austin's (2000) *Earth Spirituality*, are available for spiritually uplifting storytelling.

### Creating New Organizing Patterns

Sometimes new care delivery organizations are put in place specifically for a spiritually oriented purpose. One such trend is parish nursing, nursing care delivery tied to a traditional religious organization. Creation of the parish nurse role has blended two notions: renewed spirituality and advanced independent nursing practice. Unfortunately, parish nursing often occurs at the lower end of the pay scale, renewing, skeptics might say, the age-old notion that nursing is a devotion to be pursued without consideration of material reward. Nevertheless, most parish nursing programs are paid positions, not volunteer work. That is, a parish nurse is hired by a religious group to tend to its parishioners or, in some cases, to its geographic neighborhood. (Block nursing may be seen as a similar offshoot in care delivery.)

The parish nurse bridges spirituality and community health. About this resurgence, Smith (1991) says:

Parish nursing was born from the vision of Reverend Granger Westberg. Rev. Westberg worked as a hospital chaplin for many years, and his experience with nurses convinced him that they were "a national treasure." With one foot in the sciences and one foot in the humanities, Westberg believed nurses had great insight into the human condition. (p. 28)

Smith discloses four generally accepted functions of the parish nurse in the new movement: (1) health educator, (2) personal health counselor, (3) trainer of volunteers, and (4) liaison with community resources. Miskelly (1995) gives a slightly different list of functions: (1) education, (2) advocacy, (3) counseling, and (4) screening. Neither Smith nor Miskelly identifies hands-on care as a major function.

Despite the fact that a parish nurse works in the context of a religious group, her functions typically are not in themselves spiritual work but support of a structure with religious objectives.

Armmer and Humbles (1995) make the point that parish nursing is an important arm of health care in the urban African-American community because it links health care with an institution (the church) that is important in the community, one that is not perceived as difficult or hostile, as may be the case with some health care institutions:

> The establishment of health care services through an arena of trust (the church) by health care providers who worked to earn the trust of the members (African-American registered nurses) was a formula for success. (p. 67)

Another largely overlooked linkage between nursing and churches has been preserved in various African-American churches where so-called nurses, often in white uniform, take care of parishioners who may faint, suffer hysterics, or manifest other health accidents during church services. Historically, the practice probably arose in services that encouraged audience experiential phenomena. These nurses are not always registered nurses. Little about the practice has been written in nursing journals.

Parish nurses and African-American nurses assisting during services represent nursing acts in a religious setting, although not necessarily incorporating spiritual care into the nursing acts themselves. It is a matter of the setting. In a Lutheran release, Martinson (1991) quotes Westberg as saying:

> [a] parish nurse is a much-needed "high-touch" component in the increasingly "high-tech" world of health care. In fact, insurers and government agencies should be singing the praises of parish nursing because it promotes preventive medicine, which is the least expensive form of health care. (p. 2)

It appears that the linkage between a parish and its nurse is one of sympathy between the purposes of the church and nursing rather than an attempt to move nursing toward a spiritual base.

Parish nursing is not the only structure to support a spiritual objective; the older hospice movement can be seen as one that puts the value of human life first in its consideration. Although hospice programs are not usually spiritual in design, they allow space for the spiritual by honoring the dying process.

Other new structures, as mentioned earlier, are those growing holistic health centers that focus on wellness, illness, or both from the client's perspective as a whole being. These programs are spurting up across the nation, more often as reimbursement becomes the norm rather than the exception. Nontraditional practitioners as well as nurse practitioners in such centers are now in a phase of integrating into the health care system, with referrals to and from traditional health care professionals.

### Incidental Effects of New Care Delivery Structures

The predominant health care model today is one of managed care. In its enactment, managed care (originally envisioned to support both cost effectiveness and improved care delivery) often focuses on the former goal to the detriment of the latter. Hence, the complexity of the system may work against those niceties seen to foster a spiritually friendly environment, for example, calm, serenity, and security. Frustrations of care delivery often extend to interactions with the payment systems. In essence, the present infrastructure of care delivery may add to the client's frustration rather than assisting him in coping with his infirmities.

In challenging managers to foster spiritual growth for self, staff, and patient, Kerfoot (1995) summarizes three challenges for managers:

1. To keep ourselves spiritually alive as leaders and human beings
2. To fuel and brighten the spirit of the ones who work for and with us and those we serve
3. To keep and strengthen the spiritual care we provide to patients and the people we serve (p. 49).

This remains a daunting challenge for today's administrator.

## SUMMARY

The new paradigm returns nursing to a consideration of spiritual matters. Nursing has an interesting history of intertwining itself with spirituality. Indeed, nursing can trace its origins to the spirituality arising from ancient religions. Further, much of our early history concerns nurses dedicated to the profession because of a religious commitment, usually to a codified belief system in the context of a given religion.

Along the way, the religious origins of nursing were lost—some would say systematically sacrificed in the name of professionalism and the scientific world-view. Even nursing schools sponsored by religious institutions frequently failed to maintain aspects of spirituality in the curriculum of caregiving. In the practice setting, spirituality become the responsibility of the chaplain, not the nurse.

Today we face a spiritual resurgence. The forces involved in the renewed focus include: (1) a major shift in the normative world-view, that is, a change in the prevailing social paradigm by which reality is interpreted; (2) a spiritual focus in the growing self-help/self-development movement; and (3) a renewed attention to the spiritual impact (intended or incidental) of implementing new care delivery models.

## REFERENCES

Anastasi, J., Dawes, N., & Ming Li, Y. (1997). Diarrhea and human immunodeficiency virus: A possible synergy for clinical practice. *Journal of Alternate and Complementary Medicine, 2,* 163–168.

Armmer, F. A., & Humbles, P. (1995). Extending health care to Urban African-Americans. *Nursing & Health Care, 16*(2), 64–68.

Austin, L. (2000). *Earth spirituality.* [Compact disk]. Waukesha, WI: Singing Bear Productions.

Barnum, B. (2002). *The new healers: Minds and hands in complementary medicine.* Long Branch, NJ: Vista.

Bauer, J. (1982). *Alcoholism and women.* Toronto, Canada: Inner City Books.

Cox M. (2002, January 21). What every nurse needs to know about rave drugs. *Advances for Nurses (Greater New York/New Jersey), 2*(2), 17–20.

Donley, R. (1991). Spiritual dimensions of health care: Nursing's mission. *Nursing & Health Care, 12,* 178–183.

Dossey, B. M., & Guzzetta, C. E. (2000). Holistic nursing practice. In B. M. Dossey, L. Keegan, & C. E. Guzzetta, (Eds.), *Holistic nursing: A handbook for practice* (3rd ed., pp. 5–33). Gaithersburg, MD: Aspen.

Environmental Television Network (1995). *Rafting through canyons at dawn.* [Videotape]. New York: Author.

George, L. (1995). *Alternative realities: The paranormal, the mystic and the transcendent in human experience.* New York: FactsOnFile.

Gold, M. S. (1984). *800-Cocaine.* New York: Bantam Books.

Grof, S., & Grof, C. (1989). *Spiritual emergency: When personal transformation becomes a crisis.* Los Angeles: Jeremy P. Tarcher.

Hillman, J. (1996). *The soul's code: In search of character and calling.* New York: Warner Books.

His Holiness the Dalai Lama, & Cutler, H. C. (1998). *The art of happiness: A handbook for living.* New York: Riverhead Books of Penguin Putnam.

Kabat-Zinn, J. (1994). *Wherever you go there you are.* New York: Hyperion.

Kerfoot, K. (1995). Today's patient care unit manager: Keeping spirituality in managed care: The nurse manager's challenge. *Nursing Economics, 13,* 49–51.

Martinson, V. (1991, October). *Founder of parish nurse movement urges return to "high-touch" health care for a "high-tech" world* [News Release]. Park Ridge, IL: Lutheran General Health Care System, pp. 1–4.

Matthews, D. A. (1997). Religion and spirituality in primary care. *Mind/Body Medicine, 2*(1), 9–19.

Miskelly, S. (1995). A parish nursing model: Applying the community health nursing process in a church community. *Journal of Community Health Nursing, 12*(1), 1–4.

Moore, T. (1994). *Care of the soul.* New York: Harper Perennial.

Myss, C. (1996). *Anatomy of the spirit: The seven stages of power and healing.* New York: Three Rivers.

Newman, M. A. (2000). *Health as expanding consciousness* (2nd ed). Boston: Jones and Bartlett.

Peck, M. S. (1997). *Denial of the soul*. New York: Harmony Books.

Prince, R. H., & Reiss, M. (1990). Psychiatry and the irrational: Does our scientific world view interfere with the adaptation of psychotics? *Psychiatric Journal of the University of Ottawa, 15*(3), 137–143.

Rogers, M. E. (1970). *An introduction to the theoretical basis of nursing*. Philadelphia: Davis.

Rogers, M. E. (1994). Nursing science evolves. In M. Madrid & E. A. M. Barrett (Eds.), *Rogers' scientific art of nursing practice* (pp. 3–9). New York: National League for Nursing Press.

St. Luke's Episcopal Hospital Center for Innovation (Producer/Director). (1994). The Healing Spirit at St. Luke's Episcopal Hospital [Videotape]. (Available from St. Luke's Episcopal Hospital Center for Innovation, 6720 Bertner Avenue, Houston, TX 77030.)

Santoro, J., & Cohen, R. (1997). *The angry heart: Overcoming borderline and addictive disorders: An interactive self-help guide*. Oakland, CA: New Harbinger.

Smith, P. K. (1991). The parish nurse. *The Communique* (Quarterly publication of the Wisconsin League for Nursing, Inc), *2*, 28–29.

Watson, J. (1999). *Nursing: Human science and human care: A theory of nursing*. Boston: Jones and Bartlett.

Wilbur, K. (1983). *A sociable god: Toward a new understanding of religion*. Boulder, CO: New Science Library (Shambhala).

Wilbur, K. (1993). *The spectrum of consciousness* (20th anniversary ed.). Wheaton, IL: Quest Books.

Wilbur, K. (1999). *One taste: The journals of Ken Wilbur*. Boston: Shambhala.

Zukav, G. (1989). *The seat of the soul*. New York: Simon & Schuster.

Zukav, G. (2001). *The dancing Wu Li masters: An overview of the new physics*. New York: HarperCollins Perennial Classics.

# Chapter 2

## Spirituality and Nursing's History

This review of nursing's spiritual heritage will be incomplete and selective. No chapter can do justice to the whole history of nursing worldwide. Focus will be placed on those spiritually associated movements in the Western world.

Since the beginning of known time, people have always attempted to provide for each other the two functions of caring for and curing the ill. In that sense, nursing has always existed. At one time, nursing was more closely associated with the caring aspect; now, especially as nurse practitioners attain prominence in the profession, nursing must lay claim to both caring and curing functions. This means that our history also changes to include historical curing activities.

In this chapter we'll provide a very brief review of spirituality related to caring and curing activities up to the time when nursing and medicine split into two different professions/occupations. Then we'll shift, as nursing did, to the effects of spirituality specific to nursing.

### SHAMANISM

Spirituality has been linked with the curing aspect of human activities from earliest times. Indeed, almost every indigenous tribe worldwide practiced some form of shamanism linking notions of reality and health. Moreover, shamanism is making a comeback in this nation under new paradigm beliefs. We'll briefly look at the structure of shamanism as one of the most ancient links of spirituality and health. Shamanism began in a time when there was not the split between physical health and other aspects of being, so it looks quite different from the images of health that pertain in our society now.

Shamanism adheres closely to nature, where its forces (e.g., wind, sun, rain, as well as all things—plant, animal, mineral) within the environment are seen as having inherent, intelligent powers. Although its format changed from culture to culture, the basic tenets of the shamanic world are very similar.

The shamanic upper and lower worlds (above and below the earth) in each culture were accessed through a trance state that makes shamanism the first linking of altered states of consciousness with a religious world-view. Shamanic practice used knowledge of these alternate worlds for healing. The shamanic "world" opened in the trance state represents a life-view very different from the reality (or religious interpretations) in our dominant society today. Although differing from culture to culture, shamanism offers some universal themes. One concerns the three realms of reality: upper, middle (earth), and lower worlds. As Eliade (1987) describes the worlds:

> [t]here are three great cosmic regions, which can be successively traversed because they are linked together by a central axis. This axis, of course, passes through an "opening," a "hole"; it is through this hole that the gods descend to earth and the dead to the subterranean regions; it is through the same hole that the soul of the shaman in ecstasy can fly up or down in the course of his celestial or infernal journeys. (p. 17)

The central axis is sometimes described as a cosmic tree or a cosmic mountain. Most shamanic sagas tell of a break in the cosmic tree, making it impossible for ordinary people to ascend to the Sky World. Later, this catastrophe finds a parallel in the destructive flood of the Old Testament in Judaism and Christianity. One need not be a shaman to visit the upper and lower worlds, but Eliade (1987) describes the shaman as the one who knows the mystery of breakthrough passage among the three cosmic zones of earth, sky, and underworld.

The shamanic lower world reveals animals, humans, or near-human foes and allies, and various creatures who have discrete powers that may be used for good or evil. Forces are personified; for example, the North Wind would be an entity with its own goals and pursuits. Shamans, as Harner (1990) says, are (for they still exist) the last humans able to talk with the animals and the last ones able to talk with all of nature, including the plants, the streams, the air, and the rocks. Our ancient hunting and gathering ancestors, Harner notes, "recognized that their environment held the power of life and death over them, and considered such communication essential for their survival" (p. xiii). Hence, an important focus of shamanism is dealing with "spirits," that is, transpersonal forces that can bring illness or death:

> What, then, are "spirits"? Cross-culturally, "spirits" are subjectively described as those transpersonal forces that we experience as moving in us or through us but are not entirely moved *by* us. This means that

these (usually) personified forces or agencies are autonomous entities with their own agendas. Generally they cannot be contacted and engaged while we are in an ordinary state of waking consciousness, but are more clearly seen when we are in altered states. Dreams are the most common altered state in which they appear. (Eliade, 1987, p. 48)

These spirits may be employed as allies by humans who gain access to them, and typically, a shaman has one or many power animals who serve as his primary guides in the other worlds.

The shaman's work is conducted in the realm of the imagination, and their expertise in using that terrain for the benefit of the community has been recognized since the dawn of civilization. Their voyages allow them to experience the Creator, seek wisdom, and heal the ailments of the body. (Achterberg, 1987, p. 103)

Shamans learn to enter the shamanic world at will. Once there, they assess the illnesses of, and potential cures for, a client. Shamans use health practices of (1) soul retrieval in the lower world (returning parts of the self split off by traumatic occurrences), (2) restoring lost energy, and (3) extracting negative energy.

Shamanic work can be compared to health care in modern times. For example, soul retrieval closely resembles modern psychotherapy whereby the therapist seeks to find repressed portions of the client's personality. Like the psychiatrist, the shaman is very careful not to return a missing portion of "soul" that has not been cleansed of its damage. Extraction of negative energy or restoring lost energy sounds much like modern goals of energy movement systems such as therapeutic touch or Reiki. More traditionally, restoring energy has always been a part of medicine, for example, bed rest for the cardiac patient. Similarly, tranquilizers could be seen as relieving negative energy.

Harner (1990) describes the shamanic state and its entry point in the following way:

In engaging in shamanic practice, one moves between what I term an Ordinary State of Consciousness (OSC) and a Shamanic State of Consciousness (SSC). . . . The difference in these states of consciousness can perhaps be illustrated by referring to animals. Dragons, griffins, and other animals that would be considered "mythical" by us in the OSC are "real" in the SSC. (p. xix)

Shamans reach the trance state (usually a light theta trance) by various methods: ingestion of natural herbs/biologics, sustained pain, or sensory manipulations, particularly those achieved through repetitive rhythmic sounds:

Out of the body "journeys" have been reported following significant periods of sensory deprivation, sensory overload, or monotonous or repetitive stimulation—all three of which are part of the usual ritual for attaining the SSC [shamanic state of consciousness]. (Achterberg, 1987, p. 111)

The shaman's drum reigns as the most important means to enter other realities, and as one of the most universal characteristics of shamanism. . . . (Achterberg, 1987, p. 118)

Shamanic drumming, (auditory driving), maintains a repetitive and rapid beat that programs the brain for the experience of the shamanic world. George (1995) defines auditory driving in this way:

The power of sound in banishing our ordinary sense of reality is based on a direct impact of auditory stimulation on the human nervous system. This effect is known as auditory driving. (p. 21)

The electrical activity of the neurons in the brain tends to be rhythmic, as revealed in the wavelike patterns of EEG tracings. This natural pattern of activity is susceptible to influence by rhythmic sensory input; brain cells tend to fire in synchrony with repetitious sounds. (p. 22)

Modern shaman Sharon Blessum (2001) describes the world-view behind her soul retrieval work in the following way:

One major way we defend ourselves against the pain to our psyche is by *disassociating* . . . We split off, meaning that a part of us "goes somewhere else." (p. 83)

The part that goes away is part of our soul. The sound is *energy*, so it goes into the spirit world where it stays until it is safe to return. It is in the energy field and is available to be returned to us when we are ready to be whole. (pp. 83–84)

Harner's (1990) work is probably the best single source for a person interested in further tracking shamanism and its methods of health care.

**GREEK PRACTICES**

Moving forward in time from early indigenous shamanic practices, the pre-Roman mystery schools, in existence even before the Hellenic Greeks and long before Christ (Cavendish, 1989), also used trance states to achieve knowledge of the world and health care. These schools traced their origins back to early Egyptian practices. Probably the most famous was the Elusian mysteries, held at Elusis, fourteen miles west of Athens. This school was in existence as early as the 15th century BC (Cavendish). The mystery schools did not segregate notions of health from other life aspects. Like shamanic practice, these mystery schools used altered states of consciousness to achieve their goals. Cavendish claims that what was fundamental to all the mysteries, without exception, was the revelation of the enigmas of death and its triumphal overcoming.

Because these schools were cloaked in secrecy, we are not entirely certain what methods they used to induce these altered states. Unsubstantiated tales describe methods much like the modern use of psychedelics. Some propose that potentially life-threatening trials were used, bringing the experience closer to the near-death experiences of our day.

In ancient Greece, mystic rites were involved in seeking knowledge of the future as well as finding cures for illness. Seers commonly used drugs to produce the altered states of consciousness in which they would see visions. Seer positions were filled by a series of women—their use of hallucinogenic herbs probably contributing to the women being short-lived. An oracle of some importance in the Greek association of nursing and spirituality was the Oracle at Delphi (the most famous oracle throughout Greece, oracles of Dodona and Delos being less well known, at least in historical accounts). Concerning the oracle at Delphi Temple (1992) says:

> It was claimed that the sybil, or prophetess, sat on a tripod over a chasm in the earth from which intoxicating fumes (supposed to arise from the rotting corpse of a mythological monster called Python) rose up to send her into a prophetic trance. . . .
> The whole tale was probably invented as a cover-story to explain the strange smell of the intoxicating fumes from burning drug-plants. Inhaling fumes or swallowing drugs can induce states which bring visions of various kinds. (p. 70)

The use of such drug intoxicants, of course, is found in the armamentarium of shamans worldwide in any generation.

Early Greek healing involved altered patterns of consciousness in the supplicant as well as in the therapist/oracle. Patients were carefully prepared for visits to oracles through baths, fasting, and medications, including various hallucinogenics. In these preparations they frequently received healing dreams and visions. Sometimes Aesculapius, the classical God of Medicine, appeared in such visions. Aesculapius, son of Apollo, is usually portrayed holding the wand of Mercury, the caduceus entwined with sacred serpents (Sellew & Nuesse, 1951).

As early as the sixth to fourth century BC, the Greeks had goddesses who, in early nursing texts, exemplified the aims of nursing. Aesculapius was linked to four feminine figures associated with nursing: his wife Epione, the soothing one; and his three daughters, Hygeia, the Goddess of Health; Panacea, the Goddess of Healing; and Meditrina, the Goddess of Preservation of Health (Sellew & Nuesse, 1951). Early nurse historians often traced our origins to Hygeia. This retrospective association, of course, served the political purpose of separating nursing and medicine. Before that historical division, health care was certainly not on two different pathways.

Of interest in these associations is the fact that health and cure are personified as gods and goddesses, clearly linking pantheistic religion with care of the sick and the healthy as early as the sixth century BC. Placement of nursing in the mythopoetic religion of the times clearly sets the profession as spiritual or religious in origin.

It is also significant that the figures associated with nursing were female while the figures associated with medicine were male (one could include Hippocrates who came later, born 460 BC). This pattern of gender association has not been totally consistent over the ages, but more often than not, it has been present.

Another aspect of interest is the distinction between curing and preserving health. From the start, Aesculapius, associated with cure, had higher ranking than his daughters, associated with health and caring. Of course the traditional association with these lesser goddesses rather than with Aesculapius was the choice of nurse historians.

Recently, Moody (1993), an early explorer of near-death experiences, attempted, with mixed success, to use some of these ancient methods, not for healing, but to invoke visits from the deceased. For this purpose he created a modern-day psychomanteum where preparation, to a significant degree, followed ancient Greek processes. The negative press that he received for his efforts may have had more to do with the fact that he challenged modern notions of reality than with his results.

## DRUIDIC VERSUS CHRISTIAN RELIGIONS

Nor was Greece the only early civilization that could be associated with nursing, and certainly with health and illness. In the British Isles in the pre-Christian era, we find druids worshiping, not a god, but a goddess or a pantheon of gods and goddesses, often with female characteristics and a dominant fertility orientation. Not surprisingly, women held roles of preeminence in these Celtic religious rites. Druidic practices gave rise to priestesses who were expert in use of herbs in both health and, like other oracles, in forecasting and communicating with the deities.

These practices were still in place when the Christian, male-dominated religion was brought to the British Isles. In fiction, the historical duel between the ancient female-dominated druidic religion and the male-dominated Christianity was popularized in Bradley's (1982) *The Mists of Avalon.*

## EARLY ROMAN TIMES

Back in Greece, Roman dominance after the birth and life of Christ yielded another pattern linking spirituality and nursing functions. That was the conversion of many wealthy Roman women to Christianity, for example, Fabiola, St. Marcella, and St. Paula. These women adopted the Christian philosophy of service, often exercised in care of the sick. The Roman women served the Christian ideology with their not inconsequential worldly fortunes, thereby funding and founding many hospitals and hospices (Sellew & Nuesse, 1951).

It is interesting how the pattern of wealthy, educated women buoying up nursing has pertained sporadically throughout the history of nursing. This includes such people as Nightingale herself, as well as leaders such as Isabel Hampton Robb. (See Armeny [1983] for an interesting review of women philanthropists in America from 1898 to 1920.)

From the early Roman societies, on through the Dark Ages and medieval times, as Minkowski (1992) says:

> In the absence of curative medical or surgical therapies, nursing care was the preeminent service, one that offered little more than comfort in its provision of bed, board, bath, and prayer. A remarkable outburst of intellectual and socially directed energy found expression in secular nursing groups in the 12th and 13th centuries. In an age still superstitious and capable of great cruelty, nursing appealed to women's piety and compassion as well as to their striving for some measure of independence from a constricting social system. (p. 289)

## MEDIEVAL TIMES

The Medieval Age, sometimes called the Middle Age or the Dark Ages, covers a wide span of time from about 500 AD to 1450 AD. The period was characterized by the dominance of the Christian religion in the human psyche. It was typical that religious organizations were responsible for the growth of hospitals, such as they were.

> The medieval hospital was essentially an ecclesiastical facility with staggering mortality rates that encouraged a vision of cure only in the

hereafter. For that reason, therapy focused more on the soul than on the body. (Minkowski, 1992, p. 289)

Many church-initiated movements occurred during this period. Circa 529 AD, St. Benedict, who founded the order named after him, spread monasteries throughout Europe, requiring that each be equipped with something unique: an infirmary. In 542 AD, the Hotel Dieu of Lyons admitted women who served as nurses. The institution was ruled by a religious order of male rectors, but the women nurses did take vows (Pavey, 1959).

Nor should the Knights Hospitallers of St. John be ignored in looking at nursing's spiritual history. During the crusades, this order built shelters, hospitals, and monasteries along the routes of pilgrimage to Jerusalem. The Knights Hospitallers numbered men and some women among those who provided service to the sick (Pavey, 1959).

Medieval times are best remembered by the failure of all medicine in the fourteenth century Black Death. The bubonic plague (1348–1350 AD) killed about one-third of the population from India to Iceland before it faded. Of course, its relationship to the fleas and mice that were carriers was not understood at the time (Tuchman, 1978).

In medieval times, early nurses were often "fallen women" who took up care of the ill to redirect or redeem their lives. Widows who were left without resources were the other group identified by various historians as nurses. The influx of women into Christian church service grew into the deaconess movement, a movement eventually captured by the church male hierarchy. Ultimately, deaconesses could only be selected by the bishop (Pavey, 1959).

Later, in 441 AD, the First Council of Orange further constrained the position of women in the church with the edict that deaconesses could no longer be ordained. By the sixth century, they were also forbidden to marry or leave the order for any reason. After death, their private property become the property of the Church.

Notice that in medieval times, the struggle was not between medicine and nursing but between the religious ordination of nurses versus ordinated males and the subservience of the nursing orders to those males. This was a battle lost to the male hierarchy, just as the druids lost out to the Christian male-controlled religion in the British Isles.

The association of nursing and religion continued through the Christian monastic orders of the Middle Ages, the Knights Hospitallers during the Crusades, and even in long-standing orders such as the Alexian Brotherhood that came into being when the black death decimated much of Europe. Here one might note the entry of male groups into caregiving, with the Alexian Brothers and the Knights Hospitallers.

The deaconess movement was one of the few systems within the Christian religion that gave single women and widows a rare outlet in an era when few other positions of responsibility were available to women (Pavey, 1959). It was slowly but efficiently taken over by the church patriarchy. The Church Order of 533 AD confirmed this judgment that women could not be ordained, "by reason of the frailty of this sex" (Pavey, 1959, p. 106). Today, of course, within the formalized Christian church systems, we still have Protestant deaconesses and Catholic sisters (still not permitted to be ordained). These may be counterposed to the modern Wicca (witchcraft) movement, a trend that may be interpreted as a move back to times when religions, and the roles of women as leaders in them, were not constrained.

Margot Adler, author of *Drawing Down the Moon* (1979), claimed that the modern Wicca movement (as well as various other groups of witches, druids, and goddess worshipers) probably owe their very existence to the Church and its major restriction against women's serious participation. Like the older pagan religions, the modern Wicca movement (white witchcraft) is not devoted to health interests per se but often is involved in healing processes.

All of this is not to ignore the important role played by the Christian religion in nursing and health care through the ages. Indeed, Christianity was the first religion to take care of the ill as an important spiritual charge.

Today, of course, we have remnants of nursing orders associated with religious sects. Various Roman Catholic orders as well as the protestant Deaconess movement come to mind.

## NIGHTINGALE

The history of nursing has often been treated as if it began with Nightingale. Indeed, many assert that Nightingale was the beginning of *professional* nursing. Yet, as we have reviewed, we can claim a lengthy history before Nightingale's time, and most of those beginnings were tied to the dominant form of religion of the times. On the whole, however, in the age of a rational paradigm, we simply forgot these roots and traced our origins to Florence Nightingale, the mother of modern nursing. Modern, of course, indicates an escape from the thrall of religion into science.

### Impact of Nightingale on Nursing Spirituality

This book does not attempt to provide a history of Nightingale. Rather, it looks at those spiritual aspects of her life. For a more comprehensive review of Nightingale's life see: Macrae, 2001; Pavey, 1959; Schuyler, 1992; Sellew & Nuesse, 1951; Vicinus & Nergaard, 1990.

As is always the case, any era reflects its particular interests by the history of those it selects as significant. For decades Florence Nightingale was cast in a scientific/scholarly image: Nightingale the environmentalist, the administrator, the founder of schools, the statistician, and even Nightingale the nurse theorist.

We might note that by Nightingale's time, with the growth of medicine, there was already the bifurcation between medicine and nursing, healing and caregiving. Nightingale, a crusader in other aspects, never questioned the nurse's subservience to the physician.

Few nurses know that Nightingale had a spiritual side. Cook (1923) says that she wrote frequent meditations and occasionally heard "the voice." An Anglican who flirted with Catholicism, Nightingale was impressed with the works of Catholic sisters and with many aspects of the Catholic religion, but not enough to convert. She resisted the kind of obedience she felt the Catholic church required of its members (Vicinus & Nergaard, 1990).

Nightingale's correspondence often dealt with spiritual matters, and many of her comments sounded more New Age than the typical Anglican or Catholic orthodoxy of her era. For example, she wrote:

> Heaven is neither a place nor a time. There might be a heaven not only *here* but *now*. It is true that sometimes we must sacrifice not only health of the body but health of mind (or peace) in the interest of God; that is, we must sacrifice heaven. (Cook, 1923, p. 233)

In many ways Nightingale's comment reminds one of Newman's (1994) contemporary stance that disease is not necessarily bad but may be a signal of growth, repatterning, and expanding consciousness—the latter notion Newman's equivalent of spiritual growth.

### Mysticism

Many of Nightingale's thoughts about spiritual matters might be better classified as mystical rather than traditionally religious. She appeared to appreciate the difference between religious ritual and mysticism when she wrote:

> For what is Mysticism? Is it not the attempt to draw near to God, not by rites or ceremonies, but by inward disposition? (Cook, 1923, p. 233)

Nightingale's conception of God uses the language of mysticism through the ages. She says:

Where shall I find God? In myself. That is the true Mystical Doctrine.
But then I myself must be in a state for Him to come and dwell in me.
This is the whole aim of the Mystical Life. (Cook, 1923, p. 233)

Notice how this perspective is unlike the more plebeian religious notion
of God as some benevolent father in the sky, looking down on, but separate
from, man. For Nightingale and mystics of any century, man either is a part
of God or holds God within.

Macrae (2001) confirms this perspective of Nightingale as a mystic:

For Nightingale, spirituality is not an intellectual belief, but an actual
experience. Saying "I believe in God" is different from saying "I feel
the divine presence in my life." She felt that experience, rather than
belief by itself, is the transformative element. (p. 21)

So interested was Nightingale in mysticism that she began writing a book
on the Christian mystics of the fourteenth century. As Nightingale said of these
mystics:

These old Mystics who we call superstitious were far before us in
their ideas of God and of prayer (that is our communion with God).
(Cook, 1923. p. 234)

Peculiarly, Nightingale, who never dropped any project once she set her
teeth into it, allowed herself to be interrupted in writing her book on mystics.
After her father's death, she never returned to it.

## Life of an Invalid

After her early work in Scutari during the Crimean War, Nightingale completed most of her remaining and significant work from her home. If one thinks
about her life at the time, an interesting hypothesis comes to mind.
Nightingale's life was primarily limited to her own chambers where she held
court determining what petitioners would be admitted. This gatekeeping even
included her own family members who, like the others, required approved
appointments.

Nightingale's chief contact with the world was the written word. In
essence, she lived in a world of the mind with few infringements from the "real
world" beyond. Most acts in her world were one-on-one conversations; she
preferred to see her select visitors one at a time. Although her world was highly
limited by these tactics, one can imagine that so were the frustrations enter-

ing it. Yes, there were intellectual frustrations, but she didn't have to call a plumber for a rusty pipe, she didn't have to worry about paying the rent, and she didn't have to put up with a boss who found fault with her performance.

The world of the invalid, as Nightingale structured it, was in many ways convenient. The limited and regulated communications gave her high control and saved her from many of the normal stresses and strains others faced. Within this protected environment, Nightingale was very effective in making things happen. But, again, it was a peculiar sort of action, all through the written word and messages carried by her delegates.

One could say that Nightingale had a life with few unwanted interruptions or irritations. This is not to say that invalidism was necessarily her choice; it may simply be that she made the best of a poor situation. There are various tales concerning what malady she may have suffered, but no definitive accounts of Nightingale's physical indisposition.

Along with this sheltered environment, she had continuous adulation from those few permitted into the inner sanctum, and she had the satisfaction of seeing things get done, even if only through reports and agents.

Whatever the truth of Nightingale's personal history, this much we know: an intense zeal to promote nursing and an equal passion for spiritual development coincided in the same woman. Later generations may have chosen to ignore her spiritual side and its importance to Nightingale, but this does not alter the known fact that both elements (nursing and spirituality) consumed her interest.

### MODERN LINKAGES

Nightingale's system formed the basis for early nursing schools in the United States. Some were run by religious organizations and bore an overlay of the given church; some were secular. Reverby (1987), who documented nursing's history from 1850 to 1945, characterized the relationship of spirituality and nursing of that time this way:

> As with the middle-class man of character, behavior rather than piety became the measure of a moral being. In a woman, however, it was altruism rather than individuality that defined her moral state. (pp. 50–51)
>
> The hospital equivalent of ministers' sermons on woman's role was the physician's speech, frequently made at nursing graduation exercises. Endless homilies about loyalty and paeans to the moral good of deference sent the nursing student into her occupational world. (p. 51)

Reverby gives a remarkable review of the era that led to and began the professionalization of nursing. This period covers the shift from a religious orientation, to a moral one, and finally to a scientific orientation in which spirituality in most guises was not a dominant theme.

Yet as late as the mid-fifties, in my own early nursing career, I recall many older nurses who had been drawn to nursing as a spiritual calling, one that represented, in their era, a choice of service versus marriage and family. These women are gone now, but my memories of them are vivid. Some were dedicated to nursing with a fervor we seldom see today; others were bitter because those coming after them could "have it all" rather than choosing. On the whole, this was a remarkable group of women, caught—as we all are—in the values and patterns of their particular generation.

## SUMMARY

Of most interest to me were the spiritual leanings of Florence Nightingale. In our *interpretation* of Nightingale, we show the first real split between nursing as a spiritual calling and as a science/profession. Contrast the two dominant images of Nightingale: the lady with the lamp and the sanitary engineer and politician. Yet Nightingale herself embodied both the spiritual and the professional. Today we are moving into an era in which interest is being renewed in the spiritual motivation of Nightingale (see Macrae [2001] for example). This change in historical interest signals a paradigm shift in which spiritual values are once again attaining prominence.

## REFERENCES

Achterberg, J. (1987). The shaman: Master healer in the imaginary realm. In S. Nicholson (Compiler), *Shamanism* (pp. 103–124). Wheaton, IL: Quest Books.

Adler, M. (1979). *Drawing down the moon*. Boston: Beacon.

Armeny, S. (1983) Organized nurses, women philanthropists, and the intellectual bases for cooperation among women, 1898–1920. In E. C. Lagemann (Ed.), *Nursing history: New perspectives, new possibilities* (pp. 13–45). New York: Teachers College Press.

Blessum, S. (2001). *Luminous journeys: Natural portals to the spirit world*. USA: Xlibris (online).

Bradley, M. Z. (1982). *The mists of Avalon*. New York: Ballantine Books.

Cavendish, R. (Ed.). (1989). *Encyclopedia of the unexplained*. London: Arkana.

Cook, E. T. (1923). *The life of Florence Nightingale*. Vol. II: 1862–1910. London: Macmillan.

Eliade, M. (1987). Shamanism and cosmology. In S. Nicholson (Compiler), *Shamanism* (pp. 17–46). Wheaton, IL: Quest Books.

George, L. (1995). *Alternative realities: The paranormal, the mystic and the transcendent in human experience.* New York: FactsOnFile.

Harmer, M. (1990). *The way of the Shaman.* San Francisco: Harper SanFrancisco.

Macrae, J. A. (2001). *Nursing as a spiritual practice: A contemporary application of Florence Nightingale's views.* New York: Springer.

Minkowski, W. L. (1992). Women healers of the Middle Ages: Selected aspects of their history. *American Journal of Public Health, 82*(2), 288–295.

Moody, R. (with Perry, P.) (1993). *Reunions: Visionary encounters with departed loved ones.* New York: Ivy Books.

Newman, M. A. (1994). *Health as expanding consciousness* (2nd ed.). New York: National League for Nursing Press.

Pavey, A. E. (1959). *The story of the growth of nursing: As an art, a vocation, and a profession* (5th ed.). London: Faber & Faber.

Reverby, S. M. (1987). *Ordered to care: The dilemma of American nursing, 1850–1945.* Cambridge, England: Cambridge University Press.

Schuyler, C. B. (1992). In F. Nightingale, *Notes on nursing: what it is and what it is not* (pp. 3–17). (Commemorative edition, with commentaries by contemporary nurse leaders). Philadelphia: J. B. Lippincott.

Sellew, G., & Nuesse, C. J. (1951). *A History of nursing* (2nd ed.). St Louis: C. V. Mosby.

Temple, R. (1992). Consulting the oracles: The classic systems of Greece and Rome. In J. Matthews, (Ed.). *The world atlas of divination* (pp. 65–73). London: Bulfinch Press Book.

Tuchman, B. W. (1978). *A distant mirror: The calamitous 14th century.* New York: Ballantine Books.

Vicinus, M., & Nergaard, B. (Eds.). (1990). *Ever your, Florence Nightingale: Selected letters.* Cambridge, MA: Harvard University Press.

# PART II

## Spirituality and the Emerging Paradigm

In the beginning of this book spirituality was described as a person's search for, or expression of, his connection to a greater and meaningful context, whether that connection be with God, finding one's place in the universe, or searching for a greater sense of self. Physics, philosophy, and psychology are three domains in which that search for such meaning is conducted in three different ways: in the physical universe (physics), in the wisdom and truth underlying all disciplines (philosophy), and in the meaning of being human (psychology). Together, these three disciplines are pathways to meaning. Their goals are consistent, but their findings develop and change. The fourth domain that deals with spirituality—religion—differs from the three exploring fields in that it thinks the search is complete. Each religion is relatively certain of the correctness of its viewpoint, and has committed that belief to a codified system of worship and behavior. Religion will be addressed in chapter 12. Here, we'll look at the three domains that struggle with the eternal search for wisdom and knowledge about our reality.

Part II examines new theories from the disciplines of physics, philosophy, and psychology through the eyes of spirituality. Chapter 3 focuses on the changing world of physics, with shifts in vision from older Newtonian physics to newer quantum mechanics. Then the chapter examines changes in philosophy due to new research in physics as well as research into nonmaterial or spiritual realms as reported by subjects in altered state of consciousness. Last, the chapter includes psychological shifts that interpret and reinterpret the meaning of self.

Chapter 4 examines the meaning of the human being in his growth and development. It extends our knowledge from the more traditional developmental theories normally taught to nurses to those with transpersonal elements that incorporate spiritual growth as a natural human stage of development. Many of these theories blend Eastern and Western psychology with growth and development patterns.

# Chapter 3

## Spirituality, Physics, Philosophy, and Psychology

This chapter looks briefly at the relationship of spirituality to physics, philosophy, and psychology. Much of the emerging paradigm shift originates in the changes in these fields. Each of these disciplines represents a distinct search for ultimate meaning—in the universe, in our means of deriving wisdom, and in the human being himself.

### SPIRITUALITY AND PHYSICS

Physics hunts for meaning by understanding our universe, from the cosmic to the subatomic. At one stage, the findings of physics seemed to indicate a world—to use the most common image—that was like a clock: wound up, then left to tick away on its own. In this image, the one that predominated when Newtonian physics ruled, any notion of God the Creator was as a distant force who put things into motion, then withdrew. Humans were left to cope with the eternal laws that ruled the universe. One could use those rules, but he could not change them. Indeed, the human being was not a part of either the rules or of the God that made them.

Then physics entered the world of subatomic particles and discovered that the old Newtonian physics did not apply. In this world beneath the surface, man found that he *did* matter, that his very inquiry into it shaped the nature of the world. New discoveries in physics substantiated a complex view of reality, one that might be characterized as congruent with many of the earlier ideas of Eastern religious traditions. It was a world that called for a new reconciliation between physics and spirit. As Capra (1983) said concerning his book:

> The purpose . . . is to explore this relationship between the concepts
> of modern physics and the basic ideas in the philosophical and reli-

gious traditions of the Far East. We shall see how the two foundations of twentieth-century physics—quantum theory and relativity
theory—both force us to see the world very much in the way a
Hindu, Buddhist, or Taoist sees it, and how this similarity strength-
ens when we look at the recent attempts to combine these two theories in order to describe the phenomena of the submicroscopic
world: the properties and interactions of the subatomic particles of
which all matter is made. (pp. 4–5)

In the same spirit, Talbot (1981) discusses the fallacy of the objective/sub-
jective divisions in our world view. He opts to combine them in a single "omnijective" perception:

Indeed there is a vast philosophical and metaphysical tradition behind
the philosophy that the universe is omnijective. The mystics tell us
this is true. The idealists tell us it is true. Most exciting of all, the
physicists tell us it is true. (p. 3)

Zukav's (2001) classic work presents the clearest and most detailed explanation of modern physics for the nonphysics reader. In comparing Newtonian
physics and quantum mechanics, Zukav contrasted two realities. Newtonian
physics (the one most of us learned in school) was based on ordinary sense
perceptions. It predicted events according to scientific observations deriving
absolute rules, such as laws of motion and gravity. The rules were based on
describing things in space and time, and they allowed for calculations that
could predict events. All of this assumed an objective reality "out there," something that did not change because we observed and measured it. In contrast,
Zukav said, quantum mechanics were not observable; they described statistical behavior of systems, not of individual particles, and did not assume an
objective reality apart from our experience of it.

The new image of reality came into being when it was discovered that the
subatomic particles did not follow "common sense" Newtonian principles. We
discovered, surprisingly, that physics was not the study of metaphysics (the
study of being) so much as the study of epistemology (the study of knowing).
As Zukav (2001) said:

The new physics, quantum mechanics, tells us clearly that it is not
possible to observe reality without changing it. If we observe a certain particle collision experiment, not only do we have no way of prov-
ing that the result would have been the same if we had not been
watching it, all that we know indicates that it would not have been

the same, because the result that we got was affected by the fact that we were looking at it. (p. 33)

According to quantum mechanics there is no such thing as objectivity. We cannot eliminate ourselves from the picture. We are a part of nature, and when we study nature there is no way around the fact that nature is studying itself. Physics has become a branch of psychology, or perhaps the other way round. (p. 33)

Under quantum mechanics, notions of reality become far more complex. Take physicist David Bohm's notion of the implicate order as explained by his biographer, David Peat (interview by Alev, 1997):

Then there was his [Bohm's] theory of the implicate order. The world we seem to live in—the world of classical objects, the world of Newtonian physics—Dave referred to as the "explicate order." He felt that what we take for reality is only one particular level or perception of order. And underneath that is what he called the "implicate order," the enfolded order, in which things are folded together and deeply interconnected, and out of which the explicate order unfolds. The explicate is only, you could say, the froth on top of the milk and the implicate order is much deeper. It includes not only matter, but consciousness; it's only in the explicate order that we tend to break them apart, to see them as two separate things. (p. 27)

Explanations of physics such as this come close to what mystics have said about reality through the ages. Hence, as modern knowledge of physics grows, it serves as a bridge between spirituality and science rather than setting them at the opposite ends of the pole. Wolf (1984), claims that a shifting paradigm is long overdue and necessary to make what is taken as reality agree with the work of physicists such as Einstein, Bohm, Bell, Heisenberg, Bohr, and Planck.

A more complex world is painted by quantum mechanics, one that reveals phenomena that cannot be squeezed into the traditional scientific view. In all cases, we are forced to look anew at the similarities of world-views among physicists and mystics. Are these two disparate domains moving toward agreement? Is physics presently revealing a deep underlying core of spirituality in our reality?

## SPIRITUALITY AND PHILOSOPHY

Philosophy is the branch of study that seeks underlying wisdom and knowledge. It looks at what undergirds all of our arenas of inquiry. Hence, philosophy has many branches: Esthetics—What does it *mean* to say that something is beautiful? Logic—How do we *know* our conclusions are valid? Ethics—How do we differentiate the good from the bad, the right from the wrong?

Within philosophy, two major branches interest us in the new paradigm: metaphysics, the science of being, which asks, What really exists?; and epistemology, which asks, What does it mean to say we know? As to metaphysics, we saw that recent research in physics moved away from a philosophy of naive realism (e.g., Newtonian physics) in which the world exists out there, apart from our inquiry. In this early work, the inquiry was metaphysical in nature. Reality was seen as out there, apart from the researcher who observed it. In the new physics, however, (e.g., quantum mechanics) the thinker becomes part of the reality, and indeed his intervention in some way creates the reality. Hence we move from metaphysics toward epistemology; we see that the process of thinking constitutes or helps constitute the world. The clock maker who created the world and withdrew is no longer. We suddenly found that we were part of the creation process, indeed, part of the creator.

Kant (1986) was one of the first philosophers to recognize what has now become apparent in physics, namely, that the world is best understood through epistemology, not metaphysics, that we don't know anything directly. He says that what is "known" simply tells us how the human mind is structured rather than revealing the structure of what is "out there":

> Before objects are given to me, that is, *a priori*, I must presuppose in myself laws of the understanding which are expressed in conceptions *a priori*. To these conceptions, then, all the objects of experience must necessarily conform. Now there are objects which reason *thinks*, and that necessarily, but which cannot be given in experience, or, at least, cannot be given so as reason thinks them. The attempt to think these objects will hereafter furnish an excellent test of the new method of thought which we have adopted, and which is based on the principles that we only cognize in things *a priori* that which we ourselves place in them. (p. 7)

In this way Kant differentiated *noumena*, things "in themselves" from *phenomena*, things perceived. He clarified that we can never know the noumena directly. Moreover, the structure of our brain determines what we can learn about an object because it sets up the laws of knowing. This wisdom foresaw the direction physics would take generations later.

Certainly the changes in physics fed or complemented a changing philosophic paradigm by the shift from metaphysics to epistemology, from seeing a world "out there" to a world that was inseparable from the observer. This change in understanding created a major revision in the philosophy of science. Nursing, it might be noted, was too long wed to a philosophy of logical positivism that had a history of being associated with a world much like Newton's—out there, separate from the observer, that is, a reality that could be captured if only the right rules were applied. Years after the field of philosophy had moved on, nursing still clung to logical positivism, a situation that is now changing.

Clearly, when physics shifted its explanations of reality to epistemology (how the observer operates), there was a realization that science was speaking much like mystics of all centuries. Capra (1988) gives us an insight into how at least one physicist, Heisenberg, reacted to this growing confluence:

> In 1929 Heisenberg spent some time in India as the guest of the celebrated Indian poet Rabindranath Tagore, with whom he had long conversations about science and Indian philosophy. This introduction to Indian thought brought Heisenberg great comfort, he told me. He began to see that the recognition of relativity, interconnectedness, and impermanence as fundamental aspects of physical reality, which had been so difficult for himself and his fellow physicists, was the very basis of the Indian spiritual traditions. (p. 43)

In addition to changes in philosophy due to research by physicists, there was another group of investigators asking the big questions concerning the nature of reality. While the physicists drew conclusions from experiments, primarily with subatomic particles, these investigators went directly to the human mind, in the form of altered states of consciousness. We might label the resultant discoveries as spiritual philosophy.

These investigators were typically psychologists who used different research tools, namely hypnotic regression and out-of-body exploration. (The next section of this chapter looks at past life regression as it affects the individual in his present life, but here we will look at attempts to use altered states of consciousness to find out something about existence on different planes or levels other than earthly life.) In these explorations, humans, rather than the physical universe, became the source to be observed. The tool for exploring man was an altered state of consciousness. The most common state was the trance produced in hypnosis. When that state is achieved, the subject can be regressed to remember experiences outside of the present life.

A second state of altered consciousness was the out-of-body experience (OOBE). Subjects able to achieve this state can frequently learn to direct their encounters to an envisioned goal. As in the case of the regressed subjects, these people also can bring back what they learned in the altered state.

One of the first questions asked of these subjects concerned reincarnational past lives. However, when that narrow personal focus was played out, larger questions were posed, beginning with: What can be said about existence between lives? Work such as that of Whitton, and Fisher (1986) filtered into the market. Newton, PhD and hypnotherapist (1994, 2000) and Monroe, founder of the Monroe Institute for education and research in expanded consciousness (1985, 1994) would begin the task of detailing the afterlife and other noncorporeal "places."

Both Newton and Monroe describe hierarchies of souls clustered into groups or larger entities. Newton (1994), who used hypnotic regression, said:

> My impression of the people who believe we do have a soul is that they imagine all souls are probably mixed into one great congregation of space. Many of my subjects believe this too, before their sessions begin. After awakening, it is no wonder they express surprise with the knowledge that everyone has a designated place in the spirit world. When I began to study life in the spirit world with people under hypnosis, I was unprepared to hear about the existence of organized soul support groups. I had pictured spirits just floating around aimlessly by themselves after leaving Earth.
>
> Group placement is determined by soul level. After physical death, a soul's journey back home ends with debarkation into the space reserved for their own colony, as long as they are not a very young soul or isolated for other reasons. . . . The souls represented in these cluster groups are intimate old friends who have about the same awareness level. (p. 87)

Similarly, Monroe (1985), who helped subjects achieve various OOBEs, describes souls spinning off what he calls the Innerstate at stations determined by soul levels and belief biases. He reports finding afterlife groups of like-level souls who were committed to particular pre-death visions of heaven. For example, during an out-of-body experience, he visited a woman who had attached herself to a post-life church group similar to that which she knew in life, a group that met her expectations for heaven. She tells Monroe that periodically a soul just disappears from their group, and she doesn't know where it goes. This principle is repeated in numerous other circumstances in which a soul goes where it can, based on its maturity and understanding of afterlife existence. In his later work (1994), Monroe, along with his other-life explorers, describes and plots out large numbers of domains to which one might travel with the right trance induction.

Both Newton and Monroe interpret earth life as a school environment. Monroe (1994), who calls Earth a predator system, says:

The Earth Life System, for all its shortcomings, is an exquisite teaching machine. It brings into focus for each of us in our own way a wide understanding of energy, and the control and manipulation thereof, that is generally unavailable except through a structured environment such as time-space. The Earth Life System is a set of tools, and we learn to use them. (p. 83)

It is interesting to contemplate whether, if all its traumas and tragedies were removed, Earth would be an easier, but less efficient, learning environment for soul growth. Newton (1994) also sees Earth life as a learning environment, carefully chosen for specific soul development:

The soul must now assimilate all this information and take purposeful action based upon three primary decisions:
• Am I ready for a new physical life?
• What specific lessons do I want to undertake to advance my learning and development?
• Where should I go, and who shall I be in my next life for the best opportunity to work on my goals? (p. 202)

As Newton regressed more people, his understanding of the complexity of souls grew. For example, Newton (2000) said:

The energy of the soul is able to divide into identical parts, similar to a hologram. It may live parallel lives in other bodies although this is much less common than we read about. However, because of the dual capability of all souls, part of our light energy always remains behind in the spirit world. (p. 2)

The ability of a soul to unite with itself is a natural process of energy regeneration after physical death. A client emphatically told me, "If we were to bring 100 percent of our energy into one body during an incarnation, we would blow the circuits of the brain." A full charge of all the soul's energy into one human body would totally subjugate the brain to the soul's power. (p. 117)

More similarities than differences were seen in subjects in Newton's and Monroe's studies, despite the differences in their methods of acquiring knowledge. Newton regressed subjects by hypnosis and asked them to remember life between their reincarnations, whereas Monroe used primarily his own and others' direct experience under purposefully contrived altered states of consciousness (OOBEs).

The general flow of hypnotic regression research by all researchers was virtually predictable. Beginning with the Bridie Murphy case, researchers initially examined the concept of reincarnation (e.g., Stevenson, 1966; Weiss, 1992, 2000) and the effects of past lives on the present one. Then studies like that of Newton and Monroe began to ask questions concerning life between life, that is, research on existence outside of the body and the past or present earth lives. This research delved into the places of the soul, as one might say—the afterlife, or more exactly, the in-between life. It is not surprising that the next sort of regressive research asked yet a larger question. Modi, MD and board-certified psychiatrist (2000), asked: What can regressed people remember of God and creation?

As in the cases of Newton and Monroe, Modi found much consistency among subjects' reports. Her patients describe God this way:

According to my hypnotized patients, God is a big golden orb of energy. The center of God is very dense and the Light there is intensely bright and iridescent. As you move from the core to the periphery of God, my patients report the Light is still golden but more porous and not as dense or as intense. God is a creative energy force that grows, generates, and is constantly in motion. (p. 21)

Concerning creation, Modi's patients give similar descriptions. Here is a short portion of a summary of an early phase in the disbursal:

Before releasing the energy to create the universes, God, through Its intent, first created protective pathways, like tunnels, all over Its globe. Patients described them as similar to "spokes of a wheel," "pathways," "tunnels," "channels," or "rays" such as you see around the sun. Groups of energy swirls of similar vibrations were released through these channels out of the edge of the globe of God in a protective sac, so they would not be lost in the void. Some of these groups remained close to the ball of God, while others went further away. Sections of God in between tunnels automatically became godheads and later were programmed for their special purposes.

Patients described the energy swirls in each group, after leaving the globe of God, as clumping together in a ball and beginning to expand and contract. . . . The energy in each ball . . . continued to expand and grow and created galaxies. (p. 57)

Researchers such as Newton, Monroe, and Modi have done all they can to apply normative scientific methods. For example, they carefully script their work so that the subjects are not given suggestions as to what they should find, and they test for areas of agreement and disagreement among subjects. Monroe's investigators also try to bring back data that can be verified on deceased spirits met in their astral travels. Despite their careful collection of data, none of these regression and altered-state researchers can bridge the issue of whether the findings describe a reality apart from the subjects or, as Kant theorized, merely the structure of the human brain. The fact that the individual subjects, almost without exception, are convinced of the reality of their experience, does not change that conundrum.

Thus, while physicists continue to seek reality in the physical universe, those who work with altered states of consciousness seek to capture it in the human mind. Are these paths leading to the same conclusions? Because spirituality is concerned with ultimate meaning, these contemporary research programs inevitably affect the tenor of spirituality today. On the whole, it appears that all of these searches drive in the direction of many Eastern religions and often give results compatible with findings of mystics of all ages.

## SPIRITUALITY AND PSYCHOLOGY

In psychology, the whole notion of what it meant to be a human being changed under the new paradigm. More obviously, the person became part of the creative process—or as mystics have said in the past—man is a part of God.

Once reality became closely associated with the observer, as many said, physics became psychology. This was one of the greatest shifts in psychology: the enfolding of physics within its label. Reality became focused on the human being, his thoughts, emotions, and growth.

Another great change in psychology was the promulgation of growth and development models that reach beyond those normally taught in this country, growth and development that now extended to spiritual development as well. Because these models will be discussed at length in chapter 4, this trend will be omitted here, but the reader should keep in mind that this was one of the major new paradigm trends in psychology.

Another major change in psychology was the addition of past-lives therapy to psychotherapy. Obviously, this addition assumes an acceptance of some notion of reincarnation as reported by subjects. Here we see an Eastern concept showing up in Western world research. From this perspective, it was logical to think of humans as souls extending through time and temporarily housed in human bodies.

Regression to past lives became an avant-garde therapy for resistant psychological problems. As physician-psychiatrist Weiss (1992) says when looking at troubled relationships:

When the search for the root of the problem or its treatment is
expanded beyond the limited time span of the current relationship,
much suffering can be minimized, or even avoided. Often, the anger,
hatred, fear, and so many other negative emotions and behaviors man-
ifesting in the current life relationship may actually have had their
beginnings centuries ago. (p. 81)

In relation to hypnotic regression, there is always the issue of whether an
altered state of consciousness leads to a psychological world (just in one's
head) or a "real" world that exists in some sense external to the perceptions
of any given person.

Among new paradigm followers, a new sort of psychology appeared on
the scene to complement and sometimes challenge Freudian, Jungian, and other
extant modes of psychology. Transpersonal psychology, as Wilber (1986, 1996)
describes it, deals with the psychology of the human being who has passed
beyond the personal realms to the psychic, subtle, and causal realms. These
levels of development (discussed in chapter 4) occur at a higher level than personal levels such as achievement and self actualization, which we usually think
of as capping the development process. In the transpersonal realms, one moves
beyond the self-absorbed focus. Wilber makes a point that the transpersonal
realms may be misinterpreted by psychologists or psychiatrists who are working within traditional models (e.g., Freudian) that apply at a lower level of
development. For example, Wilber (1996) says:

They thus assume that every time there arises a consciousness not
exclusively bound to history, ego, time, or logic, the person involved
must be regressing into presocial and preegoic worlds, overlooking
the fact that the person might, just might, be contacting transtempo-
ral and transegoic truths. These critics would be forced by their very
reasoning, to the conclusion that Christ must have been hallucinat-
ing, Lao Tze was psychotic, Buddha was schizophrenic, and so with
Plato and Hegel, Aurobindo and all. (p. 214)

Grof and Grof (1989) offer a countervailing warning that treating everything as spiritual is as risky as treating everything as mental breakdown:

It is extremely important to take a balanced approach and to be able
to differentiate spiritual emergencies from genuine psychoses. While
traditional approaches tend to pathologize mystical states, there is the
opposite danger of spiritualizing psychotic states and glorifying pathology or, even worse, overlooking an organic problem. (p. xiii)

Changes in psychology inevitably are following from new definitions of the human being and his relationship to the world.

## CHANNELING

Many of the mass market books on spiritually related systems use yet another method of access to transpersonal realms—an old method revisited: channeling. Channeling is a method whereby a discarnate being temporarily "borrows" the voice of an agent (channeler) to convey a vocal message.

Edgar Cayce (Carter, 1990), known as the sleeping prophet, was probably the most famous American channeler. In recent years his fame has been partially eclipsed by Jane Roberts ((1975, 1977, 1986, 1988) channeling an entity named Seth, who dictated numerous books through her. Some channelers, like Cayce and Roberts, have little memory of what is said by the channeled entity during a session. Recordings of some sort must be made. Other channelers are able to maintain their own consciousness intact while the discarnate entity speaks.

The long list of channeled works by Roberts renewed an interest in messages from discarnate beings. Certainly Seth provided one of the more consistent world-views offered by channeling, again fostering a new interpretation of reality. The Seth literature might be heavy reading for the general population, but the easier channeled matter by the supposedly discarnate being, Ramtha, (Ramtha & Mahr, 1985), has achieved major popularity despite the serious challenges to its credibility.

Nor is vocal channeling the only route. The popular channeled books by Ruth Montgomery (e.g., 1982, 1986, 1999), are produced on the computer by the technique called automatic writing, whereby a discarnate entity takes over control of the typing. Material produced by Walsch (1995, 1997, 1998, 1999, 2000), which purports to be a direct conversation with God, is delivered by the same mcechanism, in his case in handwriting. Here is a sample of God's conversation as recorded by Walsch (1995):

> All human actions are motivated at their deepest level by one of two emotions—fear or love. In truth there are only two emotions—only two words in the language of the soul. These are the opposite ends of the great polarity which I created when I produced the universe, and your world, as you know it today. (p. 15)

Channeled materials present unique problems of validation. Ultimately the material, as many channeled entities agree, must be judged by its usefulness, whether it "feels right," and by its internal consistency. It is not easy to determine the source of channeled materials, be it beings from elsewhere (let alone whether they are wise or foolish), some dissociated part of the channeler's mind, or even whether it is out-and-out fraud. The quality of the published channeled material varies radically, but even the best of it offers no means for scientific validation.

## SUMMARY

This chapter has focused on three ways of seeking meaning: physics, philosophy, and psychology. Many of the recent findings in these areas point to the limitations of the prevailing paradigm. Indeed, many new findings are more consonant with some of the spiritual trends of the New Age. The changing world-view from the domain of physics rests in "hard science" while other fields may reflect data from less secure sources, particularly reports from subjects in altered states of consciousness.

Much of the material gives testimony to the limited scope of knowledge accessible under the scientific, traditional model. Are there other paths to knowledge? This is a major question for the new paradigm.

## REFERENCES

Alev, S. (1997, Spring/Summer). F. David Peat on David Bohm, Krishnamurti and himself: Look for truth no matter where it takes you. (Interview). *What is enlightenment?* (pp. 17–29, 84–87).

Capra, F. (1983). *The Tao of physics* (2nd ed.). New York: Bantam New Age Books.

Capra, F. (1988). *Uncommon wisdom: Conversations with remarkable people.* New York: Bantam Books.

Carter, M. (Ed.). (1990). *Four complete books: Edgar Cayce, modern prophet.* New York: Gramercy Books, Random House.

Grof, S., & Grof, C. (Eds.) (1989). *Spiritual emergency: When personal transformation becomes a crisis.* Los Angeles: Jeremy P. Tarcher.

Kant, I. (1986). *Philosophical writings* (E. Behler, Ed.) New York: Continuum.

Modi, S. (2000). *Memories of God and creation.* Charlottesville, VA: Hampton Roads.

Monroe, R. A. (1985). *Far journeys.* Garden City, NY: Doubleday.

Monroe, R. A. (1994). *Ultimate journey.* New York: Doubleday.

Montgomery, R. (1982). *Threshold to tomorrow.* New York: Fawcett Crest.

Montgomery, R. (1986). *Herald of the New Age.* New York: Fawcett Crest.

Montgomery, R. (1999). *The world to come.* New York: Harmony Books.

Newton, M. (1994). *Journey of souls.* St. Paul, MN: Llewellyn Publications.

Newton, M. (2000). *Destiny of souls: New case studies of lives between lives.* St. Paul, MN: Llewellyn Publications.

Ramtha & Mahr, D. J. (1985). *Ramtha: Voyage to the new world: An adventure into unlimitedness.* New York: Fawcett Gold Medal.

Roberts, J. (1975). *Adventures in consciousness*. New York: Bantam Books.

Roberts, J. (1977). *The "unknown" reality* (Vol. 1). Englewood Cliffs, NJ: Prentice Hall.

Roberts, J. (1986). *Dreams, "evolution," and value fulfillment* (Vol. 1). Englewood Cliffs, NJ: Prentice Hall.

Roberts, J. (1987). *Dreams and projection of consciousness*. Walpole. NH: Stillpoint.

Stevenson, I. (1966). *Twenty cases suggestive of reincarnation*. Charlottesville, VA: University of Virginia Press.

Talbot, M. (1981). *Mysticism and the new physics*. New York: Bantam Books.

Walsch, N. D. (1995). *Conversations with God: An uncommon dialogue: Book 1*. New York: G. P. Putnam's Sons.

Walsch, N. D. (1997). *Conversations with God: An uncommon dialogue: Book 2*. Charlottesville, VA: Hampton Roads.

Walsch, N. D. (1998). *Conversations with God: An uncommon dialogue: Book 3*. Charlottesville, VA: Hampton Roads.

Walsch, N. D. (1999). *Friendship with God: An uncommon dialogue*. New York: G. P. Putnam's Sons.

Walsch, N. D. (2000). *Communion with God*. New York: G. P. Putnam's Sons.

Weiss, B. L. (1992). *Through time into healing*. New York: Simon & Schuster.

Weiss, B. L. (2000). *Messages from the Masters: Tapping into the power of love*. New York: Warner Books.

Whitton, J. L., & Fisher, J. (1986). *Life between life*. New York: Warner Books.

Wilber, K. (1986).The spectrum of psychopathology, In K. Wilber, J. Engler, & D. P. Brown (Eds.), *Transformations of consciousness* (pp. 107–126). Boston: Shambhala.

Wilber, K. (1996). *Eye to eye: The quest for the new paradigm*. Boston: Shambhala.

Wolf, F. A. (1984). *Star wave: Mind, consciousness, and quantum physics*. New York: Macmillan.

Zukav, G. (2001). *The dancing Wu Li masters: An overview of the new physics*. New York: HarperCollins Perennial Classics.

# Chapter 4

## Developmental Theories:
## Is There A Spiritual Phase?

This chapter examines developmental theories, some of which propose stages of human experience beyond the usual terminal phases such as ego integrity or self-actualization. Not all developmental psychologists describe spiritual phases, but some perceive human development extending into rarefied paths, to a greater understanding of life and incorporation of its meaning into one's life trajectory. For some developmental psychologists, the higher stages might best be termed humanistic; for others, however, the characteristics are decidedly spiritual.

Many New Age nursing theories assimilate spiritual elements based on developmental schemes, and these stages of development involve some sense of expanded consciousness that may or may not be interpreted as spiritual in nature.

### MASLOW VERSUS ERIKSON

In nursing literature, Maslow and Erikson are the most frequently cited developmental psychologists. Their differences are more dramatic than their similarities. Maslow explored expanded consciousness and experiences bringing intense meaning to the experiencer. Erikson did not allow for such experiences. Both psychologists, however, described man as traversing a predictable, identifiable series of developmental stages. Erikson's classic work, *Childhood and Society* (1985) identified "eight ages of man" and described the major developmental task in each of these ages. Erikson defined his tasks by contrasting successful and unsuccessful outcomes.

The infant's task is to develop basic trust rather than mistrust. The three tasks of childhood are to develop autonomy versus shame and doubt, initia-

51

tive versus guilt, and industry versus inferiority. Four of the eight tasks of life, as defined by Erikson, are completed before the child reaches adolescence.

Erikson's task of adolescence is to acquire identity versus role confusion; then the young adult strives for intimacy versus isolation. The next phase, generativity versus stagnation, corresponds with the adult's reproductive years but is not limited to human reproduction. The rest of life is completed with a final, single task: establishing ego integrity instead of despair.

It is not surprising that the early works of many developmental psychologists deal with the early stages of life rather than the later ones. Yet many of these theorists come to recognize the existence of enhanced complexity in later life stages, often when they themselves reach those stages.

Even when he was older and studied people at the far end of the life scale, Erikson's final life phase research documented only the single developmental task: establishing ego integrity versus despair. In *Vital Involvement in Old Age* (Erikson, Erikson, & Kivnick, 1986), Erikson interviewed 29 octogenarians who had participated in his ongoing longitudinal studies. The behaviors ascribed to these subjects might be summarized as looking backward and concluding. No new modalities of perception, no new spiritual perspectives, were involved. Erikson's view of the final life phase was not encouraging:

> The future of these long-lived generations will depend on the vital involvement made possible throughout life, if old people are somehow to crown the whole sequence of experience in the preceding life stages. In other words, a life-historical continuity must be guaranteed to the whole human life cycle, so that middle life can promise a vivid generational interplay, and old age can offer what we will describe as an existential integrity—the only immortality that can be promised. (Erikson, Erikson, & Kivnick, 1986, p. 14)

Erikson's tone in describing man's final phase was even bleaker in the 1985 "afterthought" in the foreword to the re-edition of *Childhood and Society*. Here he described man in his eighties as one who

> prefers to look back and to see what summary claims, hopes, and fears have been underlined by the course taken in middle life. In old age one acquires something of a historical, and, in fact, "life-historical" identity reflecting the specific times and spaces which one has shared with one's important companions, one yet develops a—sometimes desperate—need to experience something of an existential identity encompassing one's own singular existence. (1985, p. 7)

As Erikson described it, old age is fraught with the possibility, perhaps even the likelihood, of failure to achieve that integrity which he posed as the final life phase task. Even successful achievement of integrity did not sound like a cheerful accomplishment in his description.

Erikson's (1985) portrayal of the "average" mature person did not resemble the self-actualized one described by Maslow's more pleasing picture of aging and maturing. Erikson's man was trying to "hold together"; Maslow's attempted to expand. Erikson's notion was a solemn one: "acceptance of one's one and only life cycle as something that had to be and that, by necessity, permitted of no substitutions" (p. 268).

Maslow (1970) struck a contrasting tone when he described self-actualization, saying, "What a man *can* be, he *must* be" (p. 46). For Maslow, the person actualizes his potential, reaching forward, anticipating joyfully; Erikson's subject looks backward, gathers in, perhaps with satisfaction but not necessarily with elation.

Part of the difference between Maslow and Erikson may lie in contrasting life philosophies, yet part of the difference also may rest with the nature of the human subjects they studied in reaching their conclusions. Erikson focused on "average" persons in the assorted age groups, whether or not they had been successful in their lives. Maslow, in contrast, chose to look at those who had achieved personal and professional success rather than those who failed or even become average people.

Like Erikson, Maslow's (1970) theory started with the infant. Maslow identified loosely serial needs (rather than developmental tasks) of man, beginning with physiological needs, then safety needs, needs for love and belongingness, esteem needs, needs for self-actualization, needs or desires to know and understand, and aesthetic needs.

Maslow's needs did not form a rigid hierarchy like Erikson's developmental tasks. Nevertheless, an unmet, lower-level need could assume priority for the individual, influencing the time and attention given to higher-order needs. Indeed, higher-level needs might not materialize if lower-level needs were unfulfilled. For some persons, need emergence could be atypical, reordered from the norm. The most common reversal was the emergence of self-esteem needs before needs for love and belongingness (1970).

Erikson searched for the normal experience of older people; Maslow studied those people who successfully met lower needs and moved on to higher needs. In examining self-actualizers, Maslow identified those so labeled by others or themselves. Sometimes he took exemplars, in other cases, those identified as "the healthiest" of a group, for example, his study of the "healthiest" college students. Maslow looked at these self-actualized subjects to see what they shared in common.

In Maslow's exploration of self-actualizers, he discovered what he termed "Being values" and "peak experiences." Being values involved various states of self-transcendence or mystical experience. A peak experience involved a qualitative jump in which the perception (e.g., of music, of an event, of a taste) was enhanced beyond the normal state and depth of sensation. These aspects will be described in more detail shortly. In some of Maslow's writing, Being values and peak experiences were described as modalities for self-actualization. In other instances, he agreed that they might be achieved independently of self-actualization.

### Details of Maslow's Model

Maslow's theory of human motivation proposed a flexible hierarchy in which the obstruction of lower-level needs usually inhibited a person's focus on higher-level needs. These hierarchical needs only loosely associated with the aging process in that the higher-level needs typically arose serially, when lower-level ones had been satisfied. Unlike Erikson, Maslow did not link the needs to particular age groups. His model allowed for more flexibility, with persons moving to higher-level needs based upon circumstance and achievement as much as on age.

Physiological needs predominated when all needs were unsatisfied, but their gratification released the person for the emergence of higher goals (1970). Safety needs usually arose after physiological needs and included desires for security, stability, protection, and freedom from fear, anxiety, and chaos. Safety needs embraced the desire for structure, order, and the knowledge of limits (1970).

None of Maslow's needs were irrevocably settled in a lifetime. Erikson's infant might resolve the task of developing basic trust versus mistrust early and with great permanence, but Maslow's individual could experience safety needs at any stage of development if circumstances deteriorated.

In the course of a normal life, Maslow's developing person achieved a relatively satisfactory level of safety and moved to needs for belonging and love, needs to be part of a group, and needs for intimacy. These needs, once met at a satisfactory level, gave way to needs for esteem, self-respect, mastery, and confidence in the face of the world. In addition to one's internal development of self-esteem, there was a need for esteem from others, a desire for reputation and prestige, status and recognition (1970).

Next in Maslow's hierarchy were the needs for self-actualization, that is, for self-fulfillment. In his early work, Maslow identified self-actualization by studying the "healthiest" college students and by selecting real and historical adults who were intuited to be self-actualized (1970). Cases were not focused primarily on the peak experiences or B-values that consumed so much of his later work. In his earlier work, Maslow's evidence of self-actualization included but was not limited to: (1) an ability to detect the fake, to judge people correctly; (2) an "innocent eye," the ability to live more in the world of nature than in the man-made mass of concepts, a freshness of appreciation; (3) lack of overriding guilt, shame, or anxiety; (4) good animal appetites and ability to enjoy oneself; (5) spontaneity, an ability to be unconventional without a need to flaunt the trait; (6) a focus outside of oneself, a mission in life; (7) the ability to decide for oneself, a greater sense of free will; (8) less need to cling in relations, not needing others in the ordinary sense (1970).

Later, Maslow became fascinated by what he termed, "States of Being." He categorized States of Being in many different ways, but in *The Farther Reaches of Human Nature* (1971), he described them as: (1) dealing with ends, not means; (2) creating a sense of completion, truth and reality; (3) creating a sense of perfection; (4) creating desirelessness, purposelessness due to a lack of deficiency needs; (5) metamotivational, containing the growth motivation, unmotivated by a given purpose; (6) creating a feeling of fulfillment of the self; (7) transacting with extrapsychic reality centered on the nature of the reality rather than the nature of the cognizing self; (8) transcending time and space; (9) sacred, spiritual, sublime, religious; (10) involving innocent perception; (11) reflecting ultimate holism, cosmic unity; (12) reflecting Maslow's B-values, e.g., truth and beauty; (13) resolving erst-while dichotomies by integration or transcendence; (14) creating synergic states, e.g., where opposites become equals, for example, selfishness and unselfishness assume an identity; and (15) resolving (albeit transiently) existential dilemmas, states of the human predicament (1971).

Maslow mentioned that some, but not all, self-actualizers had mystic experiences, identified then as the intensification of any experience (1970). Indeed, he differentiated between nonpeakers: practical, effective self-actualizers living in the world and doing well in it, and peakers: self-actualizers living in the realm of "Being," a realm including transcendence, symbolism, esthetics, and mystical experience (1971).

This branching seemed to indicate that suprasensory experience was not a developmental need or achievement for all persons. Maslow talked about two sorts of self-actualizers: the transcenders versus the "merely healthy" (1971, p. 283).

Between the two types of self-actualizing people, Maslow noted that, for those experiencing transcendence, the experience(s) were often central to their lives. He also granted the occasional presence of transcendent experiences among non–self-actualizers (1971) hedging on this observation by noting that such experiences are quantitatively more frequent among self-actualizers.

Maslow never doubted that transcendence happens:

> I should say also that I consider Humanistic, Third Force Psychology
> to be transitional, a preparation for a still "higher" Fourth Psychology,
> transpersonal, transhuman, centered in the cosmos rather than in
> human needs and interest, going beyond humanness, identity, self-
> actualization, and the like. (1968, p. iii)

This sort of discussion sounds very much like the transpersonal psychology that was to become popular later. Certainly these thoughts have the same
sense of the spiritual that we have used in this book. Maslow said that persons
who have peak experiences, self-transcending knowledge, might be used like
canaries in the mines, to detect realities unperceived by others:

> [I]f self-actualizing people can and do perceive reality more efficiently,
> fully and with less motivational contamination than we others do, then
> we may possibly use them as biological assays. (1968, p. 100)

With this perspective Maslow moves into spiritual development psychology. Indeed, he specifies many of the characteristics of the transcendent experience as *Being cognition:*

> In B-cognition the experience or the object tends to be seen as a whole,
> as a complete unit, detached from relations, from possible usefulness,
> from expediency, and from purpose. It is seen as if it were all there
> was in the universe, as if it were all of Being, synonymous with the
> universe. (1968, p. 74)

The B-cognition is a richer percept than the normal one; it is more fully
attended to by the percipient; it pulls him out of himself into a full absorption
in the perception:

> At the highest levels of human maturation, many dichotomies, polar-
> ities, and conflicts are fused, transcended, or resolved. Self-actualiz-
> ing people are simultaneously selfish and unselfish, Dionysian and
> Apollonian, individual and social, rational and irrational, fused with
> others and detached from others, and so on. (1968, p. 91)

The peak experience, the form in which a B-cognition presents itself, has
characteristics that identify it as "a complete, though momentary, loss of fear,
anxiety, inhibition, defense and control, a giving up of renunciation, delay and
restraint" (1968, p. 94).

Unfortunately, in nursing, attention is often given to Maslow's early work terminating in the "merely healthy" self-actualization phase. This use of his theory ignores what he considers the major thrust of his work: Being-cognition, peak experiences, and the transpersonal cosmic-centered needs he terms the Fourth Psychology.

## HUMANIST DEVELOPMENTAL THEORIES

Levinson's work, like those theories discussed earlier, dealt with stages and, in his case, plateaus of human development. Like Maslow, he focused heavily on adult phases of development, with phases consisting of pre-adulthood, early adulthood, middle adulthood, late adulthood, and late late adulthood (1977). In selecting subjects, he did not seek out the successes (like Maslow). Instead, much like Erikson, he described the patterns of both the successes and failures at various life tasks.

Levinson defined developmental stages as static planes existing between transitional periods of upheaval. Transitions have their own developmental tasks, as do the static planes. The transitional tasks differ from the static tasks in that they terminate one era and prepare for the next. These periods of rocky transition sound like normal crises, such as adolescence or mid-life crises (and one could even envision spiritual emergencies).

Although great personal change may be afoot in Levinson's transitions, they do not involve changes in the ways one thinks and feels. Instead, the person initiates new structures arising from examination of the premises and methods of the receding phase. The pattern of calm, upheaval, then calm—plateaus and transitions—may be seen as Levinson's major contribution to developmental psychology.

Levinson (1977) focused on the ways that norms and social expectations colored interpretations of human development. He stressed the social context in describing man's life structure (i.e., the patterning of an individual life at a given time). He identified numerous developmental phases for man, each with three aspects: (1) the nature of man's sociocultural world (e.g., class, religion, ethnicity, race, occupation); (2) his participation in the world (e.g., relations as worker, lover, friend, husband, father); and (3) aspects of the self (e.g., parts of self that are expressed, inhibited, or neglected).

His focus on sociology (the first two components) balanced with attention to psychology (the last component). Given the major influence of society on the individual life structure in Levinson's model, one might expect a "normal" person, sensitive to societal demands, to mask aspects of his reality that might be recognized and labeled as deviant.

R. C. Peck (1968) offered a theory of aging that built on the work of

Erikson, primarily by shifting Erikson's eight developmental tasks into the first half of life and differentiating them from additional tasks of the second half of life. Peck proposed four additional tasks for middle age and three for old age.

Middle-age tasks began with the valuing of wisdom versus valuing physical powers. Those who clung to the primacy of physical powers fell prey to middle-age depression. The second of Peck's tasks involved socializing versus sexualizing in human relationships. Here one came to regard others as persons instead of primarily as sex objects. The third task, achieving cathectic flexibility versus cathectic impoverishment, allowed for emotional versatility at a time when human relations might be shifting. Cathectic flexibility allowed one to shift investments from one person or object to another with relative ease. The final task of middle age, according to Peck, was to acquire mental flexibility versus rigidity. Failure in the last task produced a person with a set of answers to all of life's exigencies, rigid rules that created a rigid mind structure, constricting further development.

Peck's three tasks of old age were: (1) ego differentiation versus work-role preoccupation, (2) body transcendence versus body preoccupation, and (3) ego transcendence versus ego preoccupation. The first task, usually accomplished in one's sixties, involved a shift in the value system, allowing a broader range of role activities.

Peck identified the final two phases of old age as states of transcendence, but his meaning was closer to Erikson's notion of "getting through" than to Maslow's notion of "ascending beyond." For example, one either focused on the declining powers of the body or determined to simply ignore the changes and enjoy life despite them.

The last stage, ego transcendence, took place in the "certain prospect of personal death" and included providing for others who will remain, and adapting to the prospect of one's death (1968, p. 91). Peck's notion of ego transcendence called for active involvement with the future beyond the boundaries of one's mortality, yet one did not escape his own mortality in this activity. It is clear that Peck did not see "transcendence" in the sense meant by Maslow. Indeed, Peck's final transcendence closely resembled Erikson's notion of ego integrity.

Giele (1980) also spoke of the transcendence of aging in this fashion. She spoke of older persons who have the capacity to cross over age and sex stereotypes both in traits exhibited and tasks attempted. She offered exemplars such as older fathers of young children, older students, and younger college presidents. Giele's notion of transcendence involved reordering of life tasks rather than making substantive changes in the nature of those tasks or in one's perceptual modalities.

Gould (1980) also spoke of the transformations of early and middle adulthood as an expansion of self-definition. His descriptions involved shifts in thinking and feeling that fit well within the traditional paradigm for this society, that is, they involved no conscious enhancement or spiritual perception. Gould spoke of both desirable and undesirable changes, such as shifts in the defensive systems, new levels of passion for life, adopting false ideas that create barriers to growth, and linking of false ideas in a belief constellation.

Neugarten (1968) in a similar perspective spoke of

[the] heightened importance of introspection in the mental life of middle-aged persons: the stock-taking, the increased reflection, and above all, the structuring and restructuring of experience—that is, the processing of new information in light of experience; the use of this knowledge and expertise for the achievement of desired ends; the handing over to others or guarding for oneself the fruits of one's experience. (p. 139)

Erikson, Peck, Giele, Gould, Levinson, and Neugarten have values that might best be described as humanistic rather than spiritual. Maslow stands in contrast to this position by identifying transcendent values.

## TRANSCENDENT DEVELOPMENTAL THEORIES

Gowan (1974) was one of the early theorists to deal with transcendent values. Like Newman in nursing (we'll discuss her theory in chapter 9), Gowan dealt with expanded consciousness. He called the person who developed an expanded consciousness "psychedelic" and advocated promoting the conscious modification of one's belief structure to foster an expanded consciousness:

To enable us to better acceptance of unusual data, it is obviously necessary to expand our models. For experiences, like guests in a house, can be received only if the host has concepts roomy enough to accommodate them. Otherwise, as history clearly shows, they are "explained" away. (1974, p. 1)

Gowan made an important differentiation between the psychic and the psychedelic in the following way:

One important distinction between psychic and psychedelic is that psychic experiences are not developmental and psychedelic are. That is, psychic experiences may occur to the individual at any state of development but psychedelic experiences, wherein the mind-expansion occurs with some degree of rationality and control, are definitely confined to the seventh stage (generativity-psychedelia), and hence when these mystic or peak experiences occur, it is a sign that the individual's development has reached that level." (1974, p. 102)

In his differentiation between the psychic and the psychedelic, Gowan clarified an inconsistency raised by Maslow: that is, why some persons who are not self-actualized may have peak experiences and experience Being cognition. Gowan explained that the same phenomena of expanded consciousness may occur to two different sorts of persons under two different sets of circumstances.

The psychic may have instances of expanded consciousness entirely separate from his growth and development as a human being. In contrast, the psychedelic person develops these modalities of feeling and knowing as a result of and as a stage in personal growth.

Although both Maslow and Gowan proposed stages of development involving expanded consciousness, the two men differed in the nature of the phenomena that they addressed. Gowan dealt primarily, though not exclusively, with phenomena that have been termed extrasensory, such as telepathy, precognition, psychokinesis, out of body travel, clairvoyance, and perception of apparitions.

The phenomena that Maslow (1971) identified, in contrast, related more to qualitative jumps in normal modes of perceiving, changes in the nature and depth of sensations. For example, he described peak experiences as transient moments of self-actualization, as "small mystical experiences, moments of ecstasy" (p. 48). Maslow characterized these experiences within a transcendent, ontological psychology where one deals with ends, not means. Here one experiences states of anxiety-free desirelessness; states in which one experiences an ultimate holism with the cosmos; experiences that transcend time and space; spiritual states of sublime transcendence; and states in which ordinary dichotomies disappear and are integrated (1971).

Although there is no absolute discrimination possible between the experiences identified by Maslow and Gowan, Maslow's phenomena were more focused on feelings, Gowan's more on cognition. For example, a person with precognition (a Gowan-type phenomenon), might clearly predict the future occurrence of a specific event, yet a person undergoing a momentary sense of cosmic unity (a Maslow-type phenomenon) might have great difficulty expressing how his notion of reality was changed by the experience. The difference in subject matter between Maslow and Gowan is a matter of degree and preference rather than absolute. Both of them fluctuate between domains of psychic and spiritual elements. The spiritual and the psychic often blend in New Age theories.

Like Gowan, Wilber, Engler, and Brown (1986), asserted the natural development of an expanded consciousness with maturity. Theirs was an early introduction of growth and development theory that contained transpersonal levels. Although such models had long existed in Eastern philosophies, Wilber, Engler, and Brown proposed such a theory formulated for the Western mind, and at a time when new paradigm ideas were just beginning to be welcomed.

Like the others discussed here, they conceptualized human development in stages. In their investigations, they stepped across boundaries between psychoanalytic and meditative-contemplative traditions:

> Taken together these various approaches—conventional and contemplative—seem to point to a general, universal, and cross-cultural spectrum of human development, consisting of various developmental lines and stages that, however otherwise different their specific cultural or surface structures might appear, nevertheless share certain recognizable similarities or deep structures. (1986, p. 3)

These authors identified the contemplative stages of development arising after the individual has completed the stages described by Erikson and others in his tradition. They roughly divided development into the personal and the transpersonal (contemplative).

Wilber (1986) introduced life phases that explicitly dealt with mystic and transcendental phenomena. Drawing on Eastern models, his transpersonal developmental model outstripped the more traditional Western developmental models like Erikson's and Maslow's. Wilber proposed ten phases of human development, whose content is briefly paraphrased here. The stages included:

1. Sensoriphysical—sensation, perception, and sensorimotor function
2. Phantasmic—the emotional, sexual, libidinal components
3. Representational mind—preoperational thought (in Piagetian [1976] terms)
4. Rule/role mind—concrete operational thinking, with ability to take the role of the other
5. Formal-reflexive mind—formal thinking, ability to deal with the hypothetical, the reasoning mind
6. Vision-logic—dialectic, integrative networks of ideas (highest personal realm)
7. Psychic—opening of transcendental/transpersonal, contemplative developments, visionary insight reaching beyond personal concerns and perspectives

8. Subtle—seat of archetypes, platonic forms, transcendent insight, realm
   of illumination, intuition, experiences of rapture
9. Causal—universal, formless self experienced (nirvana), ego subordi-
   nated, lost in largeness of being, feelings of wide cosmic perception
10. Ultimate—absolute Spirit, radiant and all-pervading, experiences of
    "empty-suchness" (1986).

Wilber's early phases more or less equate with the work of more traditional phase theorists. It is the latter "add-on" stages that are unique. Wilber,
and others who followed in his wake, said that transpersonal development contained normal stages of growth and development, albeit phases that not everyone
achieves. Wilber's stages, beginning with the opening of the transcendental/
transpersonal (the psychic phase), all have a spiritual, mystic tone. As Wilber
(1985) says:

> As we . . . move on toward the transpersonal bands, we leave behind
> the familiarity and common sense orientations to ourselves and our
> worlds. For we are entering the world of beyond and above, where
> we begin to touch an awareness that transcends the individual and dis-
> closes to a person something that passes far beyond himself. (p. 123)

For the transpersonal psychologist, psychology becomes spiritual, with
spirit as the ultimate driving force, aspiring toward the final successful phases
of man's development. The studies of transpersonal psychologists touch on
phenomena that were "out of bounds" for generations—the study of which
would have doomed the career of the researcher/scholar for a lifetime only a
couple of decades ago. As Wilber (1980) says:

> [t]ranscendence has as its final goal Atman, or ultimate Unity
> Consciousness in only God. All drives are a subset of that Drive, all
> wants a subset of that Want, all pushes a subset of the Pull—and that
> whole movement is what we call the Atman-project: the drive of God
> towards God, Buddha towards Buddha, Brahman towards Brahman,
> but carried out initially through the intermediary of the human psy-
> che, with results that range from ecstatic to catastrophic. (p. ix)

Like Wilber, Grof's (1988) and Grof and Grof's (1989, 1990) work, primarily arising in psychology, delves into ontology (the nature of being), span-
ning the domains of physics, older psychology, and transpersonal realms. Grof
(1988) used a developmental scheme, contrasting a *hylotropic* mode of consciousness (matter-oriented, i.e., everyday) with a *holotropic* (aiming toward

the whole and characterized by nonordinary psychological states, such as meditative, mystical, or psychedelic). Among his subcategories for the holotropic realms, he also differentiated subtle and causal domains:

> Both the subtle and the causal levels can be further subdivided into lower and higher. The *lower subtle*, or *astral-psychic, level* contains traditionally out-of-body experiences, astral travel, occult and psychic phenomena (precognition, clairvoyance, psychokinesis), auras, and similar experiences. The *higher subtle level* comprises archetypal forms of deities, supreme presences and spiritual guides, experiences of divine inspiration, visions of light, and audible illuminations. The *lower causal level* is the realms of . . . the final God, creator of all the realms. . . . The *higher causal realm* is characterized by ultimate transcendence and release into boundless radiance. . . . On this level, there is no subject or object, no self or god, only formless consciousness as such. On the level of the *Absolute*, consciousness awakens to its original condition and suchness, which is also suchness of all of existence—gross, subtle, and causal. (pp. 39–40)

Thus we have models where the transpersonal realm is a natural phase of human growth and development. In these models, having achieved the earlier stages of development would lead one to these spiritual levels. Clearly, when we are talking about mystic, direct experiences with God at these high levels, we are saying that a very intense form of spirituality is a natural phase of human development.

One question that arises in these advanced phases is the fate of the ego. Both Wilber and Grof propose final stages in which the ego disappears or becomes formless. Yet, in theories of developmental maturation, this does not preclude the need for a healthy ego at lower levels. Almaas (1989) appreciates the need for normal achievement before spiritual achievement when he says (concerning spiritual development):

> It is true the individual will have to learn to let his ego boundaries dissolve and let go of his sense of individuality. But how can he let go of his sense of individuality until he knows he has one? First he will need to see that he has individuality; he has to see and understand what individuality is before he can let go of it. (p. 20)

Engler (1986) reflects the same thought in what has become a classic statement: "Put very simply, you have to be somebody before you can be nobody" (p. 24).

Wilber not only proposes stages of human development up to (or, in his terms, down to the depths of) transpersonal realms but also says there are psychological schools appropriate to each phase, with Freud aiming at persons in lower phases of development than Jung, and Jung aiming at phases less developed than later transpersonal psychology. On discussing the parting between Freud and Jung, he explained:

> [a]ny psychological researcher, investigating a particular level of the spectrum, will generally acknowledge as real all levels on and above his own, but will often deny reality to any level deeper than his own. He will proclaim these deeper levels to be pathological, illusory, or nonexistent.
>
> Freud ended up confining his remarkable and courageous investigations to the ego, persona, and shadow. But Jung, fully acknowledging these upper levels, managed to push his explorations all the way down to the transpersonal bands. Jung was the first major European psychologist to discover and explore significant aspects of the transpersonal realm of human awareness. Freud could not comprehend this, confined as he was to the upper levels, and thus the two men traveled their separate paths. (1985, pp. 124–125)

The works of Grof (1988), and Grof and Grof (1989, 1990), also go beyond the tenets set by Freud and Jung. Grof's interest is wide, ranging from prenatal and birth experiences that shape human consciousness to transpersonal realms. Grof and Grof (1990) have a special interest in what they term spiritual emergency:

> In modern society, spiritual values have been, in general, replaced by materialistic considerations and largely ignored. It is now becoming increasingly evident that a craving for transcendence and a need for inner development are basic and normal aspects of human nature. Mystical states can be profoundly healing and can have an important positive impact on the life of the person involved. Moreover, many difficult episodes of nonordinary states of consciousness can be seen as crises of spiritual transformation and opening. Stormy experiences of this kind—or "spiritual emergencies," as we call them—have been repeatedly described in sacred literature of all ages as rough passages along the mystical path. (p. 31)

## GROWTH AND DEVELOPMENT SPECIFIC TO SPIRITUAL MATURITY

The popular works of physician-counselor M. Scott Peck (1993, 1997), for example, integrate psychology with a more traditional religious perspective of Christian origin. Of course, there are those who claim that Peck's religion is not traditional at all, for example, when he says:

> [t]here are people who, at a particular point of their psychospiritual development (like alcoholics newly converted to AA, or criminals newly converted to a moral life), *need* some very clear-cut, dogmatic kinds of faiths and beliefs and principles by which to live. Nonetheless, it is my intent to tell you that the fully mature spiritual person is not so much a clinger to dogma as an explorer, every bit as much as any scientist, and that there is no such thing as a complete faith. Reality, like God, is something we can only approach. (1993, p. 79)

Peck's (1983) work admits the ontological existence of evil (as opposed to seeing it as an absence of good). Like the others discussed here, Peck breaks down traditional boundaries, in this case between psychiatry and religion, remaining within a traditional religious perspective. Like many psychologists we have already discussed, Peck (1993) identifies phases of human development, but in this case, they are phases of psychospiritual development. Stage One is antisocial, involving an absence of spirituality and unprincipled behavior that may be exerted under a pretense of being loving but is actually manipulative.

Peck labels Stage Two as formal/institutional, and it is characterized by submission to the rules of some organization—for most people, a church, temple, or mosque. Stage Three incites rebellion from unthinking submission, often resulting in doubters, atheists, and agnostics. Characterized by deep truth seeking, this stage, says Peck, is skeptic/individual, and often populated by scientists.

Stage Four lacks the formal display of religion as well as the rebellion against it. This mystical/communal stage is populated by people who have seen the cohesion beneath the surface of things—unity and community, as Peck calls it. They are happy living in mystery (1993). Interestingly, Peck says that the meaning of biblical and other religious texts will vary depending on the stage achieved by the reader.

Like Peck, Fowler (1981) also gives spiritual stages of development. A brief synopsis of his seven stages (drawn from his book on the subject) follows. Fowler associates his stages loosely with age. In brief they are: (1) undifferentiated (infancy); (2) intuitive-objective (ages 3 to 6); (3) mythical-lateral (ages 7 to 12); (4) synthetic-conventional (ages 13 to 20); (5) individuative-reflective (ages 21 to 30); (6) conjunctive (ages 31 to 40); and universalizing faith (ages 40 and over). Although this list gives more discriminations, it is not as easy to use as Peck's more terse categories.

## DEVELOPMENTAL CHALLENGES FOR THE NURSE

Although the nurse may learn any of these developmental categories, the complexity lies in caring for the patient who is at a higher level of development than the nurse. The problem that Wilber described in applying Freudian psychology to a patient at transcendental levels reveals the same issue we face here.

As a simple example take a nurse at Peck's Stage Two of religious development. Because this formal/institutional phase is characterized by submission to the rules of some church, the nurse at this level is likely to judge a skeptic who is seeking for deeper meaning at Stage Three to be lacking in religious development. The same point can be made for the other classifications. How could a nurse at Wilber's formal-reflexive fifth stage understand a patient at a subtle transcendental eighth stage? Nevertheless, knowledge of such advanced states might be the first step in understanding patients and preparing oneself for future advancement. Of course, this problem of people at very different levels of development having to interact is a very human problem, not just a problem for nurses and patients.

## SUMMARY

Expanded theories of developmental psychology lay the basis for much of the spirituality found in New Age theories in both psychology and nursing. These theories propose transpersonal states of human growth and experience, that is, states that focus on the meaning of life and existence outside the personal concerns of the individual. Typically these theories build the early components on traditional developmental theorists such as Erikson and Maslow, but create anew or build on Eastern spiritual literature in creating the higher developmental categories.

Although the works of Erikson and the early works of Maslow are still taught as the basis of developmental psychology in many nursing programs, later work by Maslow and newer work by transpersonal theorists often are not given, leaving a gap in the nurse's education.

## REFERENCES

Almaas, A. H. (1989). *The elixir of enlightenment.* York Beach, ME: Samuel Weiser.

Engler, J. (1986). Therapeutic aims in psychotherapy and meditation: Developmental stages in the representation of self. In K. Wilber, K. Engler, & D. P. Brown (Eds.), *Transformations of consciousness* (pp. 17–51). Boston: Shambhala.

Erikson, E. H. (1985). *Childhood and society* (2nd ed.). New York: Norton.

Erikson, E. H., Erikson, J. M., & Kivnick, H. Q. (1986). *Vital involvement in old age.* New York: Norton.

Fowler, J. (1981). *Stages of faith.* New York: HarperCollins.

Giele, J. Z. (1980). Adulthood as transcendence of age and sex. In N. J. Smelser & E. H. Erikson (Eds.), *Themes of work and love in adulthood* (pp. 151–173). Cambridge, MA: Harvard University Press.

Gould, R. L. (1980). Transformations during early and middle adult years. In N. J. Smelser & E. H. Erikson (Eds.), *Themes of work and love in adulthood* (pp. 213–237). Cambridge, MA: Harvard University Press.

Gowan, J. C. (1974). *Development of the psychedelic individual.* Buffalo, NY: Creative Education Foundation.

Grof, S. (1988). *The adventure of self-discovery.* Albany: The State University of New York Press.

Grof, S., & Grof, C. (Eds.). (1989). *Spiritual emergency: When personal transformation becomes a crisis.* Los Angeles: Jeremy P. Tarcher.

Grof, S., & Grof, C. (1990). *The stormy search for the self.* Los Angeles: Jeremy P. Tarcher.

Levinson, D. J. (1977, May). The mid-life transition: A period in adult psychosocial development. *Psychiatry, 2*(40), 99–112.

Maslow, A. H. (1968). *Toward a psychology of being* (2nd ed.). New York: Van Nostrand Reinhold.

Maslow, A. H. (1970). *Motivation and personality* (2nd ed.). New York: Harper & Row.

Maslow, A. H. (1971). *The farther reaches of human nature* (2nd ed.). New York: Viking.

Neugarten, B. L. (1968). Adult personality: Toward a psychology of the life cycle. In B. L. Neugarten (Ed.), *Middle age and aging* (pp. 137–147). Chicago: University of Chicago Press.

Peck, M. S. (1983). *People of the lie: The hope for healing human evil.* New York: Touchstone Book by Simon & Schuster.

Peck, M. S. (1993). *Further along the road less traveled: The unending journey toward spiritual growth.* New York: Touchstone Book by Simon & Schuster.

Peck, M. S. (1997). *Denial of the soul.* New York: Harmony Books.

Peck, R. C. (1968). Psychological developments in the second half of life. In B. L. Neugarten (Ed.), *Middle age and aging,* (pp. 88–92). Chicago: University of Chicago Press.

Piaget, J. (1976). The stages of intellectual development in childhood and adolescence. In H. E. Gruber & J. J. Vonèche (Eds.), *The essential Piaget* (pp. 814–819). New York: Basic Books.

Wilber, K. (1980). *The Atman project.* Wheaton, IL: Theosophical Publishing House.

Wilber, K. (1985). *No boundary: Eastern and Western approaches to personal growth.* Boston: Shambhala.

Wilber, K. (1986). The spectrum of development. In K. J. Engler, & D. P. Brown (Eds.), *Transformations of consciousness: Conventional and contemplative perspectives on development* (pp. 65–105). Boston: Shambhala.

Wilber, K., Engler, J., & Brown, D. P. (1986). *Transformations of consciousness: Conventional and contemplative perspectives on development.* Boston: New Science Library.

# PART III

## Spirituality and the Individual

Part III explores the intimate relationship between the individual and his spirituality. In this case, we look at the person's mind and brain, asking as we do so whether they are separate things or the same. We also look at the person's existential situation in facing disease and death.

Chapter 5 focuses on the mind and brain conundrum. However they relate to each other, what are their connections with spirituality? Here we also explore the delicate balance between psychotherapy and spirituality, looking at how the old paradigm interprets all mental disturbance as psychological. Is it possible for some such illnesses to actually be spiritual diseases? What might a spiritual disease look like?

Chapter 5 also looks at problems that may arise when a person pursues spiritual development in ways that overwhelm him and lead to a spiritual crisis. These are cases where the person's spiritual development, so to speak, has accelerated beyond his ability to handle it, creating a unique and newly recognized sort of emergency.

Chapter 6 specifies new research that connects the brain and elements of spirituality. Recent discoveries have located regions of the brain that seem to be specific for both religious and mystic experiences. Because these linkages are being made, we need to ask: Does a connection in the brain mean that spirituality is nothing more than an internal process? Is spirituality an illusion, a bodily response that has nothing to do with a greater reality or larger meaning? Does the brain's identified center for religion and mystic experiences prove that there is no God, for example? Or does it prove the opposite?

Chapter 7 deals with the person's relationship to his disease or illness.

Here such questions are asked as: Can disease be a spiritual lesson? Is disease a spiritual failure? How should we treat disease from a spiritual perspective? Why does disease exist? From early times primitive man has treated disease and spirit as related. Virtually every indigenous tribe had its shaman, bridging the world of illness and the world of spirit. Has modern man lost something valuable in denying this linkage?

Nurses inevitably care for patients having serious disabilities and those facing death. What spiritual resources can the nurse bring to bear in these situations? Clearly, her belief concerning these matters colors her care.

Mind, brain, and disease: three elements that have a major effect on one's spirituality. Part III touches on some of the important considerations.

# Chapter 5

## Spirituality and the Mind

This chapter looks at three important factors: (1) differentiating mind and brain and identifying their interactions, (2) raising issues of spirituality occurring in psychotherapy, and (3) examining illnesses due to spiritual emergence.

### MIND OR BRAIN?

In discussing spirit and the individual, it is first necessary to differentiate between *mind* (discussed here) and *brain* (explored in chapter 6). No one can really say how these two entities interact, where one ends and the other begins. Some would argue that there *is* no difference, that both mind and brain refer to the same thing. Many scientists in this society encourage this viewpoint. Indeed, the scientific paradigm takes a position that if it can't be measured, it doesn't exist.

Others believe that man has both a mind and a brain. This position is more common in the new paradigm, so we'll explore it here. If the mind is something other than the brain, then questions arise: Where is the mind? How does it interact with the brain?

Chopra (2000) proposes this relationship:

> I absolutely agree—in the long run the mind is much more primary than the brain in creating all perception. But for now the brain is our only concrete way of entering the mind. (p. 8)

It appears that mind, if it exists, works through the brain in a major way, at least while we inhabit bodies. Nevertheless, there are instances—out-of-body experiences and near-death experiences that seem to demonstrate that the mind can work apart from the brain. Persons in these states often report ver-

71

ifiable observation of things happening elsewhere than at the location of their bodies.

Chopra's (2000) perception of mind is not the usual one. He suggests a shared, "universal mind field," a domain that individuals tap with differing degrees of skill. He equates the universal mind field with God. Indeed, the universal mind field is the mind of God:

> Our whole notion of reality has actually been topsy-turvy. Instead of God being a vast, imaginary projection, he turns out to be the only thing that is real, and the whole universe, despite its immensity and solidity, is a projection of God's nature. (p. 2)

Morse (Morse & Perry, 2000) seems, at least in part, to agree with this position. He speaks about memory in this fashion:

> There is another approach to the concept of memory, one that says that memory is packaged and stored outside the human brain. By postulating that memories are stored outside the human brain, we can arrive at a coherent thoery of memory that explains the clinical data and resolves many contradictions. . . . It is not, in this theory of remote memory a system that always stores memory within the brain. Rather, it is a transmitter and receiver, communicating directly with a source of memory that exists outside the human brain. (p. 53)

Here, then, are two physicians who propose that the mind has access to data stored or existing outside of the brain. With these notions, one might envision, as Chopra does, a universal mind field, one where most people only tap the thoughts that they have contributed directly, but one to which some may have greater access. It may also be that we all have greater access to this universal mind in dream states. As to the relationship of mind to spirituality, it is no small leap to call this universal mind field the mind of God.

The more typical notion of mind is of an individual mind: one human/one mind. Here mind is usually seen as somehow enduring separate from the brain. Most would grant, however, that while alive in the body, the brain is an access point for mind.

Whether mind is seen as a shared territory or as an individual capacity, whatever the facts turn out to be, in our society we typically think of ourselves as located in our minds—not in our hearts nor in our souls. How we think becomes a measure of who we are. Seldom do we conceive of ourselves as merely functioning brains. Instinct, if not science, makes us think of ourselves as something larger and greater than a bit of brain tissue. Yet, as we'll see in chapter 6, the explanation simply may be that another part of the brain mediates out-of-body experiencing, or, we might say, trips out of the brain and directly into the mind.

In this chapter, however, we'll take *mind* to be prior to brain, possibly having access to spiritual dimensions. Mind involves how one thinks and feels from the internal perceptual sense, not as the neural synapses of one's brain.

## SPIRITUALITY AND PSYCHOTHERAPY

In light of new perceptions of human beings as spiritual, some psychotherapists have modified their interpretations of patient behaviors as well as their treatments. In chapter 1, Prince and Reiss (1990) broached the flaw in therapy that ignores the phenomenon of most importance to the patient (his own perception) simply because it fails to fit into the therapist's own world-view. These authors do not stand alone in giving the patients' perceptions serious attention. They note that many abnormal states of consciousness are given credence in other societies. Altered states of the shaman, for example, are accepted as normal by many.

Two conditions, possession and multiple personality, are usually troubled states and have always been viewed as splits in the psyche of the patient. The new paradigm world-view, however, leaves room for alternate explanations, at least in some cases. Is it possible that there are real external intrusions from other domains? To even explore such an alternative assumes a reality far more complex than the world-view ascribed under the scientific model—a model, incidentally, that has little room for spirituality, let alone alternate dimensions than our everyday world.

### Possession

Beginning with the famous psychic, Swedenborg (1979), several investigators of the hallucinations of psychotic patients have drawn similar conclusions: namely, that universal patterns undergird the phenomena reported by patients claiming to be "possessed" by demonic entities. Psychiatrist Van Dusen (1974), for example, carried out systematic inquiries in cases of psychotic persons for whom the "spirits" had become visible or audible. Van Dusen confirmed Swedenborg's claim that there were two types of spirits, low and high.

Unlike many traditional psychiatrists who ignore the content of their patients' hallucinations, Van Dusen asked patients at Mendocino State Hospital, California, if he could talk to the spirits that possessed them. He found that access was usually granted, and the entities possessing all patients were surprisingly similar: the lower spirits, stupid and malicious, seemed to find pleasure in torturing the patient, finding his weaknesses and working on them. Similar findings regarding possession by lower spirits are reported by Rogo (1987), who prefers the term *obsession*.

Along with demonic possession, one might also review patients' visions of angelic beings, although there seem to be no cases of possession by these entities. Nevertheless, one can ask if there is any possibility that such visions have an external source rather than being attributable to an internal psychological flaw. In allowing for angels and devils, one is reminded of Monroe's assertion that upon death, people who have irrevocable beliefs in certain views of heaven are drawn to places with the expected characteristics. Recall that Monroe (1985) reported finding afterlife groups of like-level souls who were committed to particular pre-death visions of heaven.

If all traditional religions have their own "turf" in the afterlife, then there must be territories that correspond to the common views of heaven and hell. If so, one might ask if some people enter those domains while still in the body, hence reporting such places and their inhabitants as real. One can imagine a person during out-of-body experiences coming in contact with these locations. Would remaining open to impressions from these locations be one possible way to account for those who see angels or demons? In the case of some of these persons, they might very well be unable to separate that domain from the one of everyday life.

If so, this would be an external, rather than an internal, cause of what appears to be a psychosis. As we said, to even consider such a proposal demands that one give credence to a more complex world-view than is possible under the scientific model.

If one gives credence to these alternate explanations for abnormal mental states, the question is what this has to do with spirituality. The alternate explanations depend not so much on the mental state of the victim, but on the idea that there are real, hierarchical spiritual levels of existence, with occasional "misfirings" in which a person, for various reasons, opens himself to levels of existence other than his own, making him vulnerable to possession by an entity from another dimension.

### Multiple Personality

Rogo (1987) notes that some cases attributed to multiple personality (or split-off sections of the psyche) may be better explained by obsession. This is not to imply that obsession is always the case in multiple personality, but that the presence of the symptoms calls for a differential diagnosis.

Treatment for the same symptoms would depend on the cause, with mental breakdowns amenable to traditional psychotherapeutic treatment, and obsession (in both multiple personality and other types of possession) better handled by exorcism. Interestingly, increased uses of exorcism, including recent use of the technique by the Pope himself (television news, February 22, 2002) are being reported.

There is yet another case that might be mentioned here: In religion and common parlance, one often hears about that "still small voice" within. Sometimes people use this phrase simply to refer to their own reflections or so-called conscience. Yet others truly believe that they hear a directive voice. Again, one may ask, Is this some internal split, another part of one's being talking to oneself? Is it some modified multiple personality? Is it the voice of God, of one's spirit guides, of angels? Or is it another form of possession? (Recall that Nightingale was one who heard such a voice.)

From the nurse's perspective, the most important aspect may be exploring with the patient the phenomenon he is experiencing before discounting it. Sometimes one can work with the patient to help him differentiate dimensions. I think, for example, of a patient who was encouraged to have a conversation with an "entity" who was threatening him. It was suggested that the patient tell the entity that he didn't belong in this reality and that he didn't have permission to enter. Whatever the explanations behind this approach, when the patient applied this suggestion, it was more effective than prior psychotherapy.

## Alcoholism

Alcoholism provides a different sort of linkage between psychotherapy and spirituality. Like diabetes, the AA program diagnoses alcoholism as a deficiency disease. In this case, the deficit is one of spirituality. The reader is referred to chapter 1 where the AA approach was described. Alcoholism is one of the few illnesses in which a spiritual element may be both cause and cure. As we said in chapter 1, Jung believed that the abuse of alcohol was a defective search for the spiritual. Alcohol, he said, was the equivalent, on a low level, of spiritual thirst for wholeness; it represented the search for union with god (Bauer, 1982). Hence, spirituality is the subject of both the deficit (the lack of it) and the prescription (the need for it).

If Jung's proposed cause (spiritual deficit) is correct, we should not be surprised that the most successful therapy, Alcoholics Anonymous (AA), grounds recovery in a relationship to a higher power. Although AA makes no attempt to link these programs to a specific religion, the notion of a higher power is taken quite literally. Mere body cure (namely withdrawal and detoxification) seldom works without the structured AA program.

## DISEASES DUE TO SPIRITUAL EMERGENCE

A unique classification of illnesses is emerging under the new paradigm: illnesses as the result of spiritual development gone awry. These cases arise when persons practicing spiritual techniques or developing along spiritual paths encounter a crisis. Grof and Grof (1989) list the following situations in which spiritual emergencies may occur: (1) the shamanic crisis, (2) the awakening of Kundalini (subtle body energies), (3) episodes of unitive consciousness (peak experiences), (4) psychological renewal through return to the center, (5) the crisis of psychic opening, (6) past-life experiences, (7) communication with spirit guides and "channeling," (8) near-death experiences, (9) experiences of close encounters with UFOs, and (10) possession states.

This is not to say that these states always create an emergency. For example, Kundalini experiences may be pleasurable for some people, while for others, such experiences can throw the body into severe pain. In describing how such crises arise, Grof and Grof (1989) note:

> The conscious world of consensus reality and the archetypal world of the unconscious are both authentic and necessary aspects of the human psyche. They complement each other, but are two separate and very different realms that should not be confused. While it is important to acknowledge both of them and respect their requirements with good discrimination, each at appropriate places and times, responding to both of them simultaneously is confusing and can be detrimental to functioning in everyday life. (p. 194)

Again, the issue may be how these states are to be treated. Grof and Grof (1989) assert that medication (e.g., long-term use of antipsychotics or tranquilizers) can interfere with and repress the emergent spiritual development. Instead they recommend a minimalist approach, beginning with various types of meditation, movement meditation, selected spiritual practices, working with dreams, drawing, painting, or keeping a diary. For more serious crises, they suggest, among other things, appropriate therapists, for example, transpersonal ones; temporarily slowing down of the spiritual development process; and possibly minor tranquilizers.

Wilber's (1985) notion that the nature and level of the therapy must match the level of the patient's development would seem to be important here. Treating a person suffering with a transpersonal crisis with Freudian psychology, for example, would be a recipe for failure.

Assagioli (1989) says that the therapist must be careful to differentiate spiritual crises from neurotic or borderline psychotic states:

To deal correctly with the situation, it is therefore essential to determine the basic source of the difficulties. . . . The symptoms observed isolatedly may be identical; but a careful examination of their causes, a consideration of the individual's personality in its entirety, and—most important of all—the recognition of his actual, existential situation reveal the different nature and level of the underlying conflicts. In ordinary cases, these conflicts occur among the "normal" drives, between these drives and the conscious "I," or between the individual and the outer world (particularly people closely related to him, such as parents, mate, or children). In the cases which we are considering here, however, the conflicts are between some aspect of the personality and the progressive, emerging tendencies and aspirations of a moral, religious, humanitarian, or spiritual character. (pp. 33–34)

As we said earlier, Grof and Grof (1989) offer a warning that treating everything as spiritual is as risky as treating everything as mental breakdown:

It is extremely important to take a balanced approach and to be able to differentiate spiritual emergencies from genuine psychoses. While traditional approaches tend to pathologize mystical states, there is the opposite danger of spiritualizing psychotic states and glorifying pathology or, even worse, overlooking an organic problem. (p. xiii)

## SUMMARY

There are several interesting linkages between spirituality and mind. First, we must consider just what mind is and how it relates to the brain. Some new paradigm thinkers, physicians among them, consider that mind and brain are separate. Indeed, some propose that mind is not located in the human being's body. All of this, of course, makes us look anew at what it means to be human. New conceptions of mind often involve a relationship with a higher power, and mind may have a unique relationship with that power.

We also examined traditional and new practices in psychotherapy as it relates to spirituality. Are some illnesses, previously attributed to mental impairments, actually attributable to outside forces arising from a more complex world? Are some mental illnesses actually problems that arise when spiritual development gets off track and turns into a crisis? Whether one accepts that such conditions exist (or potentially exist) depends on one's world-view. Is spirituality a source of problems as well as a source of comfort?

## REFERENCES

Assagioli, R. (1989). Self-realization and psychological disturbances. In S. Grof & C. Grof (Eds.), *Spiritual emergency: When personal transformation becomes a crisis* (pp. 27–48). Los Angeles: Jeremy B. Tarcher.

Bauer, J. (1982). *Alcoholism and women: The background and the psychology.* Toronto, Canada: Inner City Books.

Chopra, D. (2000). *How to know God: The soul's journey into the mystery of mysteries.* New York: Harmony Books.

Grof, S., & Grof, C. (1989). *Spiritual emergency: When personal transformation becomes a crisis.* Los Angeles: Jeremy P. Tarcher.

Monroe, R. A. (1985). *Far journeys.* Garden City, NY: Doubleday.

Morse, M., & Perry, P. (2000). *Where God lives: The science of the paranormal and how our brains are linked to the universe.* New York: Cliff Street Books, Harper Collins.

Prince, R. H., & Reiss, M. (1990). Psychiatry and the irrational: Does our scientific world view interfere with the adaptation of psychotics? *Psychiatric Journal of the University of Ottawa, 15*(3), 137–143.

Rogo, D. S. (1987). *The infinite boundary.* New York: Dodd, Mead.

Swedenborg, E. (1979). *Heaven and hell.* (Trans. G. F. Dole). New York: The Swedenborg Foundation.

Van Dusen, W. (1974). *The presence of other worlds.* New York: Harper & Row.

Wilber, K. (1985). *No boundary: Eastern and western approaches to personal growth.* Boston: Shambhala Publications.

# Chapter 6

## Spirituality and the Brain

Recent research shows that feelings of a spiritual and religious nature may originate in the right (or dominant) side of the brain, specifically in the temporal lobe and limbic system. The fact that a physiological correlate has been located brings to the forefront the issue of the reality of such experiences, namely, Is a religious or mystic experience all in the brain? Or does the fact that the brain has such a capacity indicate its ultimate connection to something greater?

The medical orientation (usually based on the older scientific world-view) tends to see the person who is extremely religious or who reports mystic encounters as ill. The medic with this mind-set looks for the "flawed" part or parts of the brain accountable for these experiences.

In this chapter, attention is given to the most dramatic case of spiritual and religious development, that is, the mystic, simply because little if any physiologic research has been done on the "normal" religious person. These appreciations, however, are known to arise in the same brain areas as those exercised by the mystic.

It is important to differentiate between what we might call a typical religious approach and an experiential religious/spiritual approach. A person at the first level may enjoy religion, believe in religion, but never have a religious experience beyond perhaps the same sort of awe and wonder that one might associate with beautiful music or a wonderful painting. In contrast, the religious/spiritual encounter is visionary in nature and opens up new depths of meaning. The latter *has* been studied and hence will be the focus of much in this chapter.

## BRAIN STRUCTURES

As we know, much cognition is controlled in one hemisphere of the brain, typically the left brain. These activities include understanding of spoken and written language, speech, and various areas of behavior, among them, handedness. This side of the brain controlling these functions is called the dominant side. In contrast, the right brain (more accurately, non-dominant brain) mediates more subtle functions such as emotions, motivation, mood, and short-term memory, as well as aesthetic and religious appreciations. Indeed, the area of the brain activated in the near-death experience has been pinpointed to a particular section of the right brain. In a small percentage of people, right and left brain functions are completely reversed, with the right side dominant.

In our common language, we tend to talk of left brain/right brain instead of talking about dominant/non-dominant sides of the brain. Because over 90 percent of adults have left brain dominance we tend to equate left brain and dominance, shorthand that is not accurate in about 10 percent of cases.

Not all civilizations are, or have been, so strongly reliant on left-brain functions as ours. For example, the Australian Aborigines, who consider themselves the original and true people, clearly use more right-brain skills. For example, they spend much time interpreting each other's dreams—and considering them as significant portents. They are able to "walk-about" over large expanses of uncharted land using only an "inner gyroscope" for finding their direction (unlike our left-brain maps). They value and develop right-brain abilities, establishing a different, intimate, and knowing relationship with their environment.

The existence of a group of people with highly developed right-brain skills makes us think in terms of different brains rather than assuming that the left-brain orientation is automatically better. Indeed, one can imagine that the ideal might be to have full development of both sides of the brain. Optimal functioning would include equal measures of values and thoughts, aesthetics and science. When the research is done, the highly religious person and the mystic will probably turn out to have greater functioning of the right brain than is common in most modern societies. Of course, a left-brain oriented society is likely to look askance at many right-brain functions, or at least to consider them unscientific and less important.

There is no reason to think of one side of the brain as good and the other as flawed. Yet in a left-brain dominant society, that is often the case. Take, for example, the following statement by Schiffer (1998), a physician and psychiatrist: "It seemed to us as if Ryan [a patient] was of two minds: one, more adult, more present in the immediate reality, and the other, immature or primitive" (p. xv).

Here we see the typical bias of a left-brain oriented society: failure to appreciate the subtle negotiation between the two halves of the brain and the need to judge good versus bad.

Some researchers propose the neural substrates of mystic and religious experience to include the limbic and subcortical networks of the brain. The limbic system is on the medial (inner) surface of the cerebral hemisphere, surrounding the upper part of the brainstem. In other words, the limbic system is a deeper structure than the cortex gray matter. Saver and Rabin (1997) describe the more extreme mystic phenomena associated with that portion of the brain in this way:

> What is peculiarly distinctive to religious experience would appear, on first inspection, to reside not in the domains of affect, language, or cognition, but in perception. It is the direct sensory awareness of God or the divine that is a quintessential mark of specifically religious experience. (p. 499)

Saver and Rabin (1997) leave room for the cosmological rather than the religious mystic encounter—a perspective that we would still see as spiritual as defined in this book:

> Ictal events of any type may be the subject of religious or cosmological explanation. Seizures are paroxysmal, riveting, and unexpected— sudden intrusions of unanticipated and often extraordinary experience into the ordinary daily flow of consciousness. (p. 500)

These researchers contend that interpretation of visions is individualized:

> Experiments demonstrate that individuals not only interpret, but also inwardly experience, the same physiologic stimuli in strikingly different ways according to the cognitive expectations they carry. (p. 500)

Hence an experiencer who was very religious would be likely to give a religious interpretation to his vision, although another experiencer might give a cosmic interpretation.

In addition to describing states that arise under religious or cosmological vision, we now have the medical testing capacity to assess with accuracy the particular status of a person's brain waves at any given time. As Hughes and John (1999) explain, different frequencies of brain waves are clearly associated with different levels of consciousness. Frequency ranges are separated into delta (1.5–3.5 Hz), theta (3.5–7.5 Hz), alpha (7.5–12.5 Hz), and beta

(12.5–20 Hz) bands. The alpha rhythm dominates in a healthy person at rest, while the faster beta band is believed to indicate corticocortical and thalamo-cortical transaction involved in processing specific information. Solving a problem, for example, would involve a beta range. The theta band reflects diminished sensory throughput to the cortex and may be manifest in drowsiness or trance states. The lower delta band is often present in sleep. These brain waves can now be measured by quantitative electroencephalography (QEEG), a technique that measures many more areas of brain electrical activity than traditional electroencephalography (EEG).

## MYSTIC VISIONS: PATHOLOGY OR NORMALITY?

Saver and Rabin fall into the medical pattern of describing experienced religious/mystic phenomena in terms that are laden with pathological connotations, describing states of depersonalization (loss of the sense of one's own reality), derealization (alterations in the sense of reality of one's external environment), and double consciousness, which they describe as "Double consciousness ('mental diplopia') auras create a simultaneous experience of persisting remnants of one's normal consciousness and of a new quasi-parasitical consciousness with a different perception of reality" (Saver and Rabin, 1997, p. 500).

These physicians find such religious/cosmic states in every sense pathologic without even considering that some of them might be momentary enhancements of being. From the "inside" the percipient might say, for example, that instead of double consciousness being "quasi-parasitical," the bilocation enabled him to double his awareness. Or that "derealization" was actually a view of a larger reality. But the authors are judging good and bad from the viewpoint of the average man. Their summary, albeit medical, is less pejorative:

> The core qualities of religious and mystical experience, assented to
> by a wide variety of psychologists of religion, are the noetic and the
> ineffable—the sense of having touched the ultimate ground of reality and the sense of the unutterability or incommunicability of the
> experience. Frequent additional features are an experience of unity,
> an experience of timelessness and spacelessness, and a feeling of positive affect, of peace and joy. We suggest that the primary substrate
> for this experience is the limbic system. (p. 500)

Begley (2001) describes a mystic encounter occurring to Dr. James Austin as he waited for a train.

> And then Austin suddenly felt a sense of enlightenment unlike any-
> thing he had ever experienced. His sense of individual existence, of

separateness from the physical world around him, evaporated like morning mist in a bright dawn. He saw things "as they really are," he recalls. The sense of "I, me, mine" disappeared. "Time was not present," he says. "I had a sense of eternity. My old yearnings, loathings, fear of death and insinuation of selfhood vanished. I had been graced by a comprehension of the ultimate nature of things." (p. 52)

The richness of meaning in this experience, the sense of something greater than the self, clearly meets our definition of spirituality. Although this is a cosmic mystic vision rather than a religious one, its spiritual nature is typical of such visions.

Most religions trace their origins to a person having mystic visions—Jesus, Muhammad, or Buddha, for example. According to Newberg, D'Aquili, and Rause (2001):

Evidence suggests that the deepest origins of religion are based in mystical experience, and that religions persist because the wiring of the human brain continues to provide believers with a range of unitary experiences that are often interpreted as assurances that God exists. (p. 129)

Experiences tend to conform to one's religious expectations. As Newberg, D'Aquili, and Rause (2001) say:

Roman Catholics, for example, can experience Jesus' presence in the most intimate and unifying way, through the sacrament of the Eucharist, which fulfills Christ's promise of union and eternal life. In the same fashion, Buddhists use meditation and other contemplative rituals to transcend their attachments to the egotistical self, and all the mortal suffering those attachments cause, and to lose themselves in the serene oneness of existence that the Buddha so eloquently described. (p. 91)

Salloway, Malloy, and Cummings (1997) link such mystic religious experiences to lesions in the temporal/limbic circuit:

Limbic and subcortical brain regions, organized into functional units, mediate fundamental functions such as memory, emotion, motivation, and mood. Limbic and subcortical systems also play a key neurobiological role in other important aspects of human experience, such as substance abuse, reward systems, and religious experience. Most neuropsychiatric disorders involve dysfunction of subcortical structures

or the limbic or paralimbic cortex. Dysfunction of temporolimbic systemic produces some of the most dramatic and challenging syndromes
of clinical medicine. (p. 313)

Notice that these accounts label most temporolimbic phenomena as dys-
functional. However, one must keep in mind that the physician authors are
only likely to see persons for whom these phenomena present problems. From
the medical viewpoint, the assumption is that a physiological cause of hyper-
religion/mysticism lies within the brain.

The brain research that relates most closely to spirituality has been focused
on two areas: (1) the near-death experience (NDE), and (2) the brain states of
meditators.

### NEAR-DEATH EXPERIENCES

A near-death experience occurs during the time a person is clinically dead,
before resuscitation brings him back. Often called the tunnel experience because
of the sense many NDEers have of moving up a tunnel, the encounter is a vital
engagement with another level of reality. The experience often enhances the
experiencer's spirituality in that it gives him a glimpse into what is usually
perceived as the afterlife. The NDE is discussed at length in chapter 7.

Researchers into NDEs locate these experiences in the nondominant,
noncognitive side of the brain. Because most NDEs take place on a medical
turf, it is not surprising that subjects for investigations are available. Morse
(Morse & Perry, 1990, 2000) identified a physiological center in the Sylvian
fissure of the right temporal lobe just above the ear that initiates the NDE.
Morse says:

> When my research team published its report on the anatomy of the near-
> death experience, we were contacted by a group of neurologists in Chile
> who had been studying the same thing. They had arrived at the same
> anatomical conclusion that we did, that near-death experiences were
> generated by neuron activity within the Sylvian fissure. . . .
>     But exactly what did that discovery mean? They were as stumped
> as we were. (Morse & Perry, 1990, p. 109)

Although Morse claims that NDEs arise in the right temporal lobe, we don't
know whether he meant the right side or the nondominant side. He speaks as
if "right side" were true for all people, but we don't know if his sample included
any NDEers with right brain dominance.

## MEDITATION STUDIES

Laurie and Tucker (1993) describe meditation this way:

> [t]rue meditation requires an emptying of the self. One closes the eyes, goes down to alpha level, and seeks the silence rather than something within or outside the self—in short, exhausting the mind as thoroughly as possible so that ideas, sounds, and sights are eliminated. . . . The stilling of the mind is the goal. (p. 86)

As indicated here, the attempt is to shut off the left-brain internal dialogue, to allow the right brain to come into dominance. This is certainly consistent with the research showing religious and mystic experience located in the right brain. Meditation is detailed in chapter 11, and the religious form of meditation (contemplation) is discussed in chapter 12.

Radiologic studies by Newberg and D'Aquili (Newberg, D'Aquili, & Rause, 2001) used a different population than the near-death studies. They recorded changes in brain function in meditators (Buddhists and Franciscan nuns) experiencing various mystic states. Unlike Morse's studies, which looked primarily at firings in the temporal lobe, Newberg and D'Aquili focused on what parts of the brain must be tuned down or shut off to allow the mystic experience to emerge. The centers that they identify as critical were diverse, namely, four association areas of the brain: the orientation association area, the attention association area, the verbal conceptual association area, and the visual association area. These areas are located in various lobes of the brain, and are not simply concentrated in one discrete site. Together these association areas normally enable a person to differentiate himself from nonself and to locate himself in space. When these orientations were blunted, the meditators in this study entered various mystic states, the greatest being a total melding with reality and loss of self, that is, cosmic consciousness (Absolute Unitary Being in the author's terms). The mechanisms by which these states were achieved are complex and related to the type of meditation used. The reader is referred to the authors' book for details.

The decreased function in the association areas of meditators was seen using single photon emission computed tomography (SPECT). This technique reveals cases of decreased blood flow, indicative of decreased activity in a given brain area. SPECT consistently showed decreased activity in the meditators' orientation areas in the posterior parietal lobe. Tamping of such normal pathways allowed nerve firings to be diverted to alternate pathways, once again through the limbic system. In the case of passive meditation, for example, Newberg, D'Aquili, & Rause (2001) state:

[w]e believe that as the meditative state deepens, and the attention area tries more intensely to keep the mind clear of thoughts, this area, in conjunction with the hippocampus, chokes off more and more neural flow. As this blockage continues, bursts of neural impulses begin to travel, with increasing energy, from the deafferented orientation area, down through the limbic system, to the ancient neural structure known as the hypothalamus. (p. 118)

In addition to single photon emission computed tomography, there are other tools that show changes in brain functioning. Included in the spectrum of now available tools are other forms of positron emission tomography (PET), low-resolution electromagnetic tomography (LORETA), electroencephalography (EEG), and quantitative electroencephalography (QEEG). As newer medical techniques appear on the scene, we'll acquire more information about the mystic's brain physiology, but that alone can never answer the question of how internal and external realities relate. Nor are we yet able to say that all mystic experiences relate to permanent or transient altered brain physiology.

Once we have achieved definitive measures of extreme states like mystic encounters, then perhaps we'll be able to refine our knowledge of more subtle states such as spiritual and religious appreciations without greatly altered states of consciousness.

## WHAT IS REAL?

The issue is *not* whether there are brain correlates with spiritual experiences, but whether the existence of a physiological correlate means that the experience is meaningless in terms of a greater reality. Morse is one of the more positive voices in this respect. He sees no contradiction between having a physiological correlate that initiates an NDE and having the experience reveal a greater reality that is "out there." As he says:

Does the fact that we know where the experience originates make it more a reflex than a spiritual experience?

We ultimately answered "no" to this questions. Like Wilder and Penfield and others who had done brain research, we now knew where in the brain a certain action took place; we didn't know why. (Morse & Perry, 1990, p. 108)

Physicians Saver and Rabin (1997) seem to agree when they say:

Religious experience is brain-based. This should be taken as an unexceptional claim. All human experience is brain-based, including scientific reasoning, mathematical deduction, moral judgment, and artistic creation, as well as religious states of mind. Determining the neural substrates of any of these states does not automatically lessen or demean their spiritual significance. The external reality of religious percepts is neither confirmed nor disconfirmed by establishing brain correlates of religious experience. Indeed, it has been argued that demonstrating the existence of a neural apparatus sustaining religious experience can reinforce belief because it provides evidence that a higher power has so constructed humans as to possess the capacity to experience the divine. (p. 498)

What is *real*? Ironically, most mystics and medics work from a shared premise of naive realism. That is, they both believe that what they see is "real." The medics find the brain alteration real; they can test for it, measure it. The mystic finds his visions real; he has seen what he's seen firsthand. Philosophers have long debated what it means to say that something is real. As we said earlier in this book, Kant (1986), stressed the difference between *noumena* and *phenomena*, explaining that everything we accept as real is actually filtered through the capacities of the receiving human mind/brain. We don't know the noumena (the thing in itself), but we do know the phenomena (the noumena interpreted). All we really know about a thing are its properties as perceived and interpreted. A modern computer technician would say that it depends on how we are programmed. The point is a simple one: that "reality" is always reality interpreted.

Newberg, D'Aquili, and Rause (2001) make this point by recognizing that the brain is our only access to reality, whether it be the reality of mysticism or the reality of the everyday world. They recognize that access to all worlds is through the brain, that no reality can be proved to exist "out there" apart from the percipient:

All knowledge, then, is metaphorical; even our most basic sensory perceptions of the world around us can be thought of an as explanatory story created by the brain. (p. 171)


## REDUCTIONISM AND HOLISM

Many modern health care professionals, including nurses, view scientific discoveries and medical progress through a rather simple notion of reality, adopting reductionism as a method of scientific inquiry. From this philosophy, the world (or any part or element of it) is best understood by taking it apart and identifying its components.

This viewpoint ignores Kant's differentiation between noumena and phenomena, taking a more direct view of reality as "out there" and separate from the perceiver. One learns the objects of reality by taking them apart and describing their smallest elements. Water, for example, is explained as two hydrogen atoms combined with one oxygen atom. Sachdev (1999) epitomizes the reductionist viewpoint:

> I support the idea that mental phenomena are caused by neurophysiological processes and are therefore features of the brain. (p. 274)

Sachdev reduces thoughts (mental phenomena) to biology (neurophysiological processes). Granted, he recognizes that his method is reductionistic:

> The underlying concept is the idea that certain things might be shown to be *nothing but* certain other sorts of things. Any attempt to understand mental processes in terms of neurophysiological processes is therefore reductionistic in spirit. The pull in science is toward a physical understanding of all phenomena, and this is what we wish to achieve for mental phenomena. (p. 274)

As he says, "Depression is nothing but decreased transmission of serotonin in the brain" (p. 274).

Alper speaks of the "God" part of the brain as an inherited gene favored for survival. Like Sachdev, his view assumes that if there's a location in the brain, then there is no correlate in a greater reality. Alper (1999) says:

> What if spirituality represents the manifestation of one of our brain's cognitive functions? As all cultures perceive reality from a spiritual perspective, is it not possible that spirituality may represent one of the ways our species processes information and consequently interprets reality? If so, it would imply that our cross-cultural beliefs in such concepts as a god, a soul, and an afterlife constitute nothing more than the products of inherited cognitions, manifestations of the particular way our species happens to process information and, therefore, to interpret reality. In such a light, God would no longer represent any real or absolute truth, but rather a cognitively generated, subjective/relative one. In essence, such a hypothesis would imply that God, as we've thus far interpreted him (as a real and absolute entity) is reduced to just another one of our species' relative perceptions, the manifestation of an evolutionary adaptation, a coping mechanism installed in us to allow our species to survive our unique and otherwise crippling awareness of death. (p. 153)

For Alper and Sachdev, mystic encounters can be reduced to neurobiology with no relationship to a larger reality. For a long time, the nursing profession employed a philosophy (logical positivism) that was also based in a reductionist pattern. This philosophy now is in competition with holistic philosophies. Several of these are reviewed in chapter 9 where nursing theories are compared.

A holistic theory of mind/brain proposed by physician Chopra (2000) differentiates between mind and brain, seeing brain as a bodily vehicle and mind as a greater entity that cannot be located in space-time, and certainly can't be located in brain tissue. The mind is a field into which one taps rather than a confined organ; mind is greater than mere biology. As we indicated earlier, Chopra proposes a universal mind field which one accesses. Notice the difference between a "smaller entities," reductionistic viewpoint and Chopra's holistic one (explaining something by reference to its participation in something greater):

> As soon as one uses the term *field*, a step has been taken into the realm of quantum reality. The brain is a thing with material structures like a cortex and a limbic system. A field is not a thing. The magnetic field of the earth exerts a pull over every iron particle, causing it to move this way or that, yet nothing visible or tangible is doing the moving. In the same way the mind causes the brain to move this way or that. (p. 217)

With this notion, one might say that the mystic has learned to tap more dimensions of the universal mind field than is true for the average person.

The reader will recall that Morse (Morse & Perry, 2000) proposes a similar holistic theory:

> My theory allocates only short-term memory to the actual workings of the brain. Short-term memory depends on electrochemical interactions in neurons. These short-term memories, as well as all sensations, thoughts, images, and motor functions of the brain are being sorted continually and processed by a portion of our brain known as the hippocampus then blended with old memories and emotions by the limbic system. Then memory is transferred to the right temporal lobe where, I speculate, it is linked to the universal patterns of energy that surround us and make up the universe. (p. 58)

In our society people often assume a reductionist position without recognizing that they are doing so. Not only religious but often antireligious interpretations of reality both assume that a brain locus precludes an external correlate "out there." With such an unstated assumption, one who believes in a given religious leader may seek to rule out a physiological correlate while the nonbeliever sees a physiological correlate as proof that the leader's visions are false. See, for example, the Internet materials by Couperus and Hackleman (1985) (http://www.ellenwhite.org/headinjury, htm) concerning the head injury of Ellen White, a historical prophet in the Seventh-Day Adventist movement. The effort in this material is to discredit her religious visions as having been caused by temporal lobe epilepsy following a head injury. The "proof" in this case takes the form of showing that she had other symptoms of temporal lobe epilepsy. The discussion illustrates that believers and nonbelievers alike tend to accept the unstated assumption that a physical source automatically discounts the validity of visions. Because both sides tacitly accepted a reductionistic viewpoint in this argument, they could only fall back on arguments concerning whether or not her visions had a physiological basis.

Simply put, most religious devotees don't want to attribute the visions of their founding mystics to physiologic sources. Certainly in this society, any visionary state associated with a medically identifiable cause is often dismissed as illusory. Yet, as we said earlier, it is logical to ask if a mystic event *could* have a physiologic correlate and *still* represent some valid perception of a greater state of reality.

There are many such disagreements concerning whether or not mystic visions demonstrate a reality that is "out there." Mystics feel that they have witnessed a larger reality, but others are divided on the issue. One could argue that neither Morse's positive nor Sachdev's negative conclusions necessarily follow from their arguments. In other words, the conclusion that there *is* (or *is not*) a greater spiritual reality cannot be determined by physiological correlates. Whatever the relationship of the brain to outer reality, there is evidence that at least some mystic experiences can be associated with specific brain locations.

Obviously, one wonders about mystics in past eras when little was known about brain function. Historically, many mystics were known epileptics, indicating at least some level of unusual brain activity. Saver and Rabin (1997) identify as likely epileptics Saint Paul, Muhammad, St. Catherine of Genoa, St. Teresa of Avila, St. Catherine dei Ricci, Emanuel Swedenborg, Vincent Van Gogh, and St. Therese of Lisieux, among others. Histories of at least some of these historical figures recount epileptic seizures.

Borchert (1994) reports, for example:

Many mystics have continually complained of poor health. St. Teresa of Avila was subject to much running water, many little birds, and a great deal of whistling in her head. Plus chronic headaches, as was

Mechthild of Hackeborn. Fainting fits, attacks of cramps, phobias, depressions—it would be possible to draw up a whole list of symptoms out of the lives of the mystics; and many of them did not live long. (p. 15)

Does every mystic have some correlated brain anomaly? Or does every mystic encounter correspond with a temporary chemical alteration in the brain?

We have many and growing studies that link spirituality and the brain. But none of them can answer the critical question of whether the brain attaches the human being to a greater reality (holism) or whether the brain merely reflects its own composite structure (reductionism).

## SUMMARY

Religious appreciation and mystic experience are thought to be processed in the right (or nondominant) half of the brain, usually in the temporal lobe and limbic system. Research is in the early stages of discovery.

Even when a physical correlate is found for religious and mystic experiences, this cannot answer questions concerning the truth or falsity of religion or conceptions of spiritual realities beyond the everyday life. In the old scientific paradigm the view was reductionistic, with an external reality denied and all experiences attributed solely to the brain. In the new paradigm, such experiences often are viewed as visionary, revealing a hidden reality external to the brain.

We have focused here on mystic experiences because this is where the present data exist. All of this leaves out the more average state of religious belief. The difference in validation is critical. The mystic knows what he knows because he has seen it firsthand; it isn't a matter of faith. On the other hand, the typical religious person believes in a given creed, not because of a personal experience but because of faith, that is, belief in the absence of proof.

## REFERENCES

Alper, M. (1999). *The "God" part of the brain: A scientific interpretation of human spirituality and God*. Brooklyn, NY: Rogue Press.

Begley, S. (2001, May 7). Religion and the brain. *Newsweek, 137*(19), 50–57.

Borchert, B. (1994). *Mysticism: Its history and challenge*. York Beach, ME: Samuel Weiser.

Chopra, D. (2000). *How to know God: The soul's journey into the mystery of mysteries*. New York: Harmony Books.

Couperus, M. (with editorial introduction by D. Hackleman.) (1985, June). The sig-
    nificance of Ellen White's head injury. *Adventist Currents*; available on Internet
    (http://www.ellenwhite.org/headinjury.htm)
Hughes, J. R., & John, E. R. (1999, Spring). Conventional and quantitative electroen-
    cephalography in psychiatry. *Journal of Neuropsychiatry and Clinical
    Neuroscience, 11*(2), p. 192.
Kant, I. (1986). *Immanuel Kant: Philosophical writings*. (E. Behler, Trans.), New York:
    Continuum.
Laurie, S. G., & Tucker, M. J. (1993). *Centering: A guide to inner growth* (2nd ed.).
    Rochester, VT: Destiny Books.
Morse, M., & Perry, P. (1990). *Closer to the light*. New York: Villard Books, Random
    House.
Morse, M., & Perry, P. (2000). *Where God lives: The science of the paranormal and
    how our brains are linked to the universe*. New York: Cliff Street Books, Harper
    Collins.
Newberg, A., D'Aquili, E., & Rause, V. (2001). *Why God won't go away*. New York:
    Ballantine Books.
Sachdev, P. (1999, Spring). Is the reduction of mental phenomena an attainable goal?
    *Journal of Neuropsychiatry and Clinical Neurosciences, 11*(2), 274–279.
Salloway, S., Malloy, P., & Cummings, J. (1997, Summer). Introduction to the neu-
    ropsychiatry of the limbic and subcortical disorders. *Journal of Neuropsychiatry
    and Clinical Neurosciences, 9*(3), 313–314.
Saver, J. L., & Rabin, J. (1997, Summer). The neural substrates of religious experi-
    ence. *Journal of Neuropsychiatry and Clinical Neurosciences, 9*(3), 498–510.
Schiffer, F. (1998). *Of two minds*. New York: Free Press.

# Chapter 7

## Spirituality, Illness, and Death

Illness, dying, and death have always been critical human experiences that invoke one's spiritual beliefs and call upon one's spiritual center. They bring pain, threats to the self and to one's existence, and fear of the unknown. They test one's belief in existence beyond the body. Illness, dying, and death place a person in existential crisis. Times of crisis always make us question why we are here, who and what we are, and the nature of our linkage to something greater than ourselves. In other words, these conditions make us seek answers concerning our spirituality.

How one faces the critical events of illness, dying, and death depends on one's strength of character and one's beliefs concerning the larger meaning of life. Different attitudes are fostered by the older scientific paradigm and the New Age paradigm. Under the scientific model, crises of illness, dying, and death are unavoidable, negative events that happen to everyone. Illness is attributed to accident or the statistical luck of the draw. Dying and death usually are seen as the end of one's existence. None of this is to denigrate the immense progress made under the scientific model, The New Age paradigm neither rejects these scientific advancements nor calls for cessation of the model. The new paradigm simply states that the scientific paradigm applies to some parts of life, not to it all. Science is seen as one quadrant of a much larger whole that comprises reality.

Those in the New Age paradigm are more likely to view illness, dying, and death as transitional states in self-development, growth that will go on after one leaves the body. That does not mean that someone undergoing these crises loses the sense of threat, fear, and anxiety. Even with positive beliefs, pain, debilitation, and death are fearful states to face. Yet the new paradigm restores a meaning to life and to the individual's existence, even in light of these circumstances. As we will see in chapter 11, beliefs in the meaning of

93

life and one's place in the process may, in themselves, make passages easier and improve health outcomes.

In this chapter, we'll consider some of the hallmark events that invoke a sense of the spiritual. Indeed, such crises may shift persons from a scientific model to a new paradigm mentality. Faced with these challenging situations, one tends to look for meaning in one's life, not in statistical odds but in a wisdom that outstrips mere science.

The place of illness, dying, and death has always been critical in the life of the spirit. From earliest times, virtually every civilization has had its shaman, bridging the world of illness and the world of spirit. And every society, ancient or contemporary, has had its way of dealing with these critical junctures in the lives of its people.

Individuals, of course, may have philosophies that differ from those of the dominant society. The nurse cannot assume any given stance on the part of a patient. Finding out the significance of these events to the patient is critical in delivering appropriate care. Further, nurses need to discover their own underlying assumptions concerning these life crises. Without such review, nurses act on the basis of their beliefs and biases, unaware of the influence these stances have on their behavior.

This chapter looks at several facets that relate illness, dying, and death to one's spirituality, namely, beliefs concerning illness and death, the relation of self to illness, and pre-death and near death encounters. These are only a few aspects of the great human journey, but they serve to remind us of its spiritual quest.

### BELIEFS CONCERNING ILLNESS

Beliefs concerning illness are as varied as the people who hold them. Yet most people in the new paradigm attribute meaning to illness. Sometimes the meaning attaches to the cause or purpose of the illness, sometimes to the way in which one faces it. Often illness is examined through the screen of self, a higher self, or God, however interpreted.

Seeing illness as a challenge, as serving some goal, puts the patient in a good position for improvement. Illness can be interpreted as positive and educative instead of entirely negative (see Newman's theory in chapter 9 as illustration). Some New Age theories subscribe to a notion that every person creates his own world. The corollary belief is that the patient creates his own illness.

Transpersonal psychologists often claim that there is a higher self with its own purposes. As Vash (1994), a quadriplegic, says:

> At a psychospiritual level, bad things may not just happen either. There may be a transpersonal design that tends to elicit experiences—adverse

included—needed for reasons it takes a long time to understand. A hypothesis that there might be overarching Purpose in life that transcends the instrumental purposes of human personalities seems reasonable to entertain. (pp. xxiii–xxiv)

Nightingale took a causative view of illness. For example, she never believed in the germ theory of causation because, as Reverby (1987) said, "in part because she refused to accept a theory of disease etiology that appeared to be morally neutral" (p. 7).

## RELATION OF SELF TO ILLNESS

Every time one's interpretation of the human self changes, the meaning of illness changes. Hence, in a philosophy of illness, one must consider not only the beliefs about illness but also the beliefs about the self. Theories of self range, at one end of the spectrum, from seeing the human being strictly as a biological unit who will live and die, to the other end of the spectrum, in which the human being is a part of the highest Source or God.

One common view of the self is as a composite of several parts, divisible or indivisible. The parts vary from theorist to theorist (e.g., a bio-psycho-social being or a person composed of body-mind-spirit). With the view of man as composite parts, there is a pattern of claiming that illness is a sign of *disharmony* among the parts. Longway (1970) started this tradition in nursing by defining illness as a failure in one's participation in God's power. Longway's nurse helped the patient regain the part that was lost God power.

More recently, Watson (1999) calls disease disharmony among the human parts of body, mind, and soul. Soul is as vulnerable to being out of agreement as are the other components of the human being. In the mind, disharmony may be psychosocial; in the body, it may be genetic or represent other vulnerabilities; in the spirit, as Watson says:

A troubled soul can lead to illness, and illness can produce disease. Specific experiences, for example, developmental conflicts, inner suffering, guilt, self-blame, despair, loss, and grief, and general and specific stress can lead to illness and result in disease. Unknowns can also lead to illness; the unknown can only be known by experience and may require inner searching to find. Disease processes can also result from genetic, constitutional vulnerabilities and manifest themselves when disharmony is present. (p. 48)

The goal of Watson's nurse is to restore harmony among the three components. (Watson's theory is explored in chapter 9.)

One problem with theories that seek the cause of illness in the person is that they lend themselves to placing blame. The most obvious cases involve lifestyle illnesses (e.g., AIDS, alcoholism, drug addiction). All too often, along with blame comes justification for punishment (by self or others). No response by self or by others is more damaging to the self than blame. Programs like AA work to dismiss this sort of blaming. Defusing blame, of course, is not meant to discount accountabililty.

Today blaming has extended beyond lifestyle addictions into everything from cancer to injuries in train wrecks. ("Your inner self did it." "You brought it on yourself subconsciously.") Blame is not a new societal perspective on illness. Where a nurse holds strong beliefs about blame, her attitude toward the patient will be punitive. Unfortunately, we have all seen nurses who act out of this motivation. Certainly the psychological environment created by blame does nothing to set the stage for restoration of power and harmony as described by Longway and Watson. Vash (1994) gives a horrendous example of such blame at work:

> During the early months of my recovery from polio, a new practical nurse said: "Oh, my dear, you must have done something terribly evil for God to have punished you this way!" (p. 11)

## BELIEFS CONCERNING DEATH AND DYING

Kübler-Ross (1969, 1975) brought to a crashing end the social silence concerning death and dying when she identified death's final stages: denial, rage and anger, bargaining, depression, and acceptance (1975). Beginning with this opening, a new honesty, a "denial of denial" infiltrated health care. People were told when they were dying instead of being lied to; a system of denial occurred under the older scientific model, primarily because the view of life after death was so bleak.

Indeed, most holding this model assumed that death was the end of the individual. In contrast, death as an inevitable part of life was more compatible with the new paradigm. Here death was usually only seen as one stage in the growth and development of the individual soul.

Today in this country we have at least three common patterns of belief concerning death. The first belief under the scientific model is that death is the end of the individual. If he continues to exist, it is in the memories people retain of him. The second model is the traditional religious view that one "goes to heaven," typically pictured as somewhere "up there" above the Earth. In this image there usually is a heavenly father, and heaven and hell associated with reward and punishment. The new paradigm belief in a sustained existence seldom resembles the traditional heavenly image. Indeed, many new paradigm visions exist concerning life hereafter. One's existence is usually seen as radically changed in ways that are difficult to anticipate.

One of the new paradigm images views the human being as primarily a system of energy and light. In that image, Da Avabhasa (1991) says of death:

> When the present body becomes too weak to go on, it is quite naturally abandoned, but the process of abandoning the body is not the destruction of the individual being. Light cannot be destroyed. Light is always conserved. Because human beings are essentially forms of Light, they continue to exist after death, but they also continue to undergo transformations. The purpose of your existence is to surrender to Light Itself, until, instead of realizing only the changes and the transformations, you have Realized Light. (p. 261)

Imminent death forces patients, their families, and caregivers to reckon with the ultimate issues of life and its meaning. Fortunately, we live in an era when discussion of imminent death, (rather than denial) is the norm.

In nursing, the hospice movement was the first major movement to cease taking death as the enemy and viewing the quality of a death as an important factor in the quality of a life. In this paradigm a "good death" is one where the patient dies with few unresolved issues, in physical, mental, and spiritual comfort.

Nurses involved in death work should be people who have worked through their own anxieties concerning death. As Karen Soto, a head nurse who works with dying patients, says in an interview (Barnum, 1996):

> Death is an inevitable part of life, and when it's illness related, it can be a very difficuilt time if the person is in an institution that does not value dying as a unique experience in life. There's only one time that the patient is going to die. For the family, that's the only time they're going to lose their mother, their father, whoever that person is in their lives. (p. 34)

One's view of death is intimately tied to one's notion of self, of reality, and of growth. In this society, we have people facing death who have thoroughly thought out a philosophy of life and those who have avoided it until faced with this ultimate challenge. Some face it with spiritual understanding, some with existential angst. Some don't face it at all, with denial holding court until the end.

## PRE-DEATH ENCOUNTERS

In addition to the process of accepting one's incipient death, some persons undergo what we might term spiritual visions. Morse (Morse & Perry, 1990) termed the visions of the dying *pre-death visions*, the term *near-death* having already been appropriated for those resuscitated after clinical deaths. Under the scientific model such visions near the time of death were simply labeled as hallucinations. Under the new paradigm, they are considered spiritual phenomena connected to an afterlife.

Those having pre-death encounters seldom live long enough to give many details concerning their experiences, but most of us have heard dying people communicate with unseen others or even tell the living of their presence. When patients report these pre-death visits, their accounts are not the rambling, confused speech that may occur in the semicomatose patient. Indeed, these "other-worldly" reports have a different ring to them.

Often these patients report that "visitors" have come for them. Many health care professionals have seen dying patients' expressions change from those of pain and suffering to those of awe and wonder. Most nurses and physicians have also experienced the commonly associated "moment of clarity" in which a patient about to die awakens from a semi-coma or confused state and suddenly becomes clear-headed. As Soto, (Barnum, 1996) describes it:

> Even patients who are responsive will experience an increase in their level of consciousness. It's when they suddenly begin to talk to their family about things important to them or when an unconscious patient suddenly responds to your request by squeezing your hand. Sometimes it's a day before the death, sometimes a shorter period right before death. (p. 36)

Moments of clarity may or may not be associated with visionary states. Often they are too brief to allow for a deep assessment by the observers. Lucid dying patients sometimes experience a few precursory "visits" before the final pre-death visit.

The visitors in these visions may be described as deceased relatives, angels, heavenly beings, or even beings of light. Often a dying person names religious figures appropriate to his religion. Sometimes, the patient having a pre-death vision describes a place rather than people. One hears things like, "Oh, it's so beautiful."

Whether visionary encounters are identical to the near-death experiences of those who survive is a question that can't be answered. Nor are the pre-death reports as lengthy as near-death reports. The pre-death visions tend to occur only a few moments before death, so time is limited. Logic dictates that the pre-death encounter is even more common than the near-death one, although not every dying person evidences or shares such a vision.

Nurses are no longer discounting pre-death visions (if they ever did) but instead are beginning to record them. More important, they are learning how to interact with a patient who is recounting such experiences. Instead of the previous tendency to discount the patient's report ("You're just imagining it."), today's nurse accepts the pre-death vision as a valid experience for the patient, whatever the nurse's own beliefs

From a spiritual perspective, pre-death visions often are taken as evidence of the continuation of life after death. The same is true of the near-death experience.

## NEAR-DEATH EXPERIENCES

Like pre-death encounters, near-death experiences were written off as hallucinations under the scientific model. Under the new paradigm, people consider whether NDEs might be exactly what most experiencers claim: visits to the afterlife. Once again, something that was seen as an illusion under the scientific model has been recast as a potentially valid spiritual encounter under the new paradigm.

Moody (1975, 1977; Moody & Perry, 1988) was one of the early researchers of the near-death experience, conducting extensive interviews of large numbers of clinically deceased, resuscitated patients, establishing a database, and producing a comprehensive description of the NDE. Following Moody, many other researchers delved into the near-death waters (e.g., Atwater, 1994; Morse & Perry, 1990, 1992, 1993; Weiss, 1992). With modern medical resuscitation techniques, they found no lack of study subjects. Morse's research on children may be the least skewed, at least in the case of the very young, who may interpret their NDEs with less cultural/societal bias.

Researchers virtually agree on the characteristics of the NDE. The phenomenon opens similar doors for most experiencers, although we acknowledge that there are two types of near-death experience: the good and the bad encounter.

### The Good NDE

The common denominators of the good journey after death include the following: (1) having a sense of being dead, (2) feeling peace and painlessness, (3) having an out-of-body experience, (4) undergoing the tunnel experience, (5) seeing people of light, (6) meeting a being of light, (7) undergoing a life review,

(8) rising rapidly into the heavens, (9) feeling a reluctance to return to earth, and (10) having a different sense of time and space (Moody & Perry, 1988). The NDE may involve any number of these aspects, but seldom all of them.

The place visited during the NDE often contains pleasing gardens or parks, places where the vegetation is more luxurious than on Earth, possibly psychedelic, but not especially alien. For most, but not all NDEers, this after life visit is populated with deceased relatives and friends. Many NDEers have a sense that they are blocked from going too far into the perceived after life location, as if there were a barrier which, once crossed, precluded a return to life. They either feel this or are told this by some authority on the other side. Many returners are challenged with a "mission" to be completed during the rest of their lives.

Whom they see and the nature of the environment may be adapted to the experiencer's cultural and religious beliefs. The figure of light is a good example, being seen as Jesus, Muhammad, or Buddha by some and as a loving nonpersonified force by others. It appears that the NDE has a universal form, but that people place different interpretations on it.

Near-death experiencers are cognizant of others' opinions. Years ago, a patient who had a near-death experience was likely to keep it to himself so that people wouldn't think he was crazy. That still happens today with patients who have never heard of NDEs. When patients know about the phenomenon, they are more open.

Today, most nurses are taught to ask every patient who undergoes resuscitation after a clinical death whether he had any unusual experiences. It's now considered good medicine to let the patient know that reports of visions are common, that he is not alone. The professional asks in a way that lets the patient feel free to talk about what happened, if anything, without programming him for an expected response. It is also important that the nurse record the NDE and that the experience not be discounted, whatever the nurse's own belief structure. The experience is an intense one for patients and very spiritual for most of them. It is important that the experience be respected.

After an NDE, most people return with a very positive attitude toward life. They tend to value life more than previously, they are more caring toward others, and they have no fear of death. The NDE tends to become central in how the experiencer lives his life, the way he acts, and what he believes. In essence, the NDE may put a person on a spiritual path.

### The Bad NDE

A small number of persons do not find themselves in the pleasant experience described above, but in a place that is terrible. Negative NDEs occur in two ways. First, some people literally feel that they descended into hell. They describe nightmarish scenes and gruesome tortures. Berman (1995) recounts a tale told to him by one interviewee:

> About this time it became clear to me that I was an amusement to these figures who were pushing me along; that my pain was their pleasure. They weren't trying to kill me, they were simply trying to make me hurt more. Then they began clawing at me and biting at me. And just as I'd get one off, it seemed as though five more would be back on me, clawing and pushing. I had the sense that there were innumerable numbers of these people clawing at me, working to make me as miserable as possible. (p. 88)

Atwater (1994) describes the hell-like cases as characterized by

> lifeless or threatening apparitions; barren or ugly expanses; threats, screams, silence; danger and the possibility of violence and/or torture; and a feeling of cold (or of temperature extremes), and a sense of hell. (p. 45)

Subsequently, experiencers of bad NDE trips tend to firmly believe in the existence of hell, and, not surprisingly, many change their behaviors because they don't ever want to return there.

The second type of negative NDE is not a trip to hell but a life review undergone by someone who has chronically abused others during his life. In the life review, a person becomes the recipient of all the feelings of pain or pleasure that he has given to others. Hence, if one spent much of a lifetime inflicting physical and emotional pain on others, he will experience all these feelings as if they were his own. A near-death experiencer, Dannion Brinkley (Brinkley & Perry, 1994) said:

> This life review was not pleasant. From the moment it began until it ended, I was faced with the sickening reality that I had been an unpleasant person, someone who was self-centered and mean. . . . Now, as I reviewed my life in the bosom of the Being, I relived each one of those altercations, but with one major difference: I was the receiver. . . . I felt the anguish and the humiliation my opponent felt. (pp. 12–13)

Like those who experienced versions of hell, those undergoing a negative life review also are motivated to change in positive ways. Both types of negative experiencers may want to change their behaviors radically while they still are living and have the opportunity.

A prior interest in spiritual matters doesn't determine who has an NDE and who doesn't. Nor does the character of the person. Indeed, the near-death experiencer may undergo phenomena that contradict his prior belief structure. Yet there are few who emerge from the experience without a new spiritual context that influences the remainder of their lives.

### Persons Not Undergoing an NDE

Not every resuscitated, clinically dead person recounts an NDE. Many say they have no memory at all for the time during which they were clinically deceased. To my knowledge, there has not yet been research done on this class of returner. One can propose many different explanations for why some resuscitated, clinically deceased persons do not have an NDE. Perhaps they simply had no such experience. It would be interesting if medical parameters could compare non-experiencers and experiencers. Even in a normal clinical death, it is difficult for medicine to set exact parameters between living and dead, short of bodily decay. Alternately, it may be that these clinically deceased persons who can't recount an NDE simply don't bring their experiences back with them, that they have forgotten their NDEs. Hypnosis might be a tool useful in seeing if any blocked memories exist for this group.

### SUMMARY

The meaning of illness, dying, and death to the individual depends on his philosophy concerning what is real, his understanding of the causes and purposes of illness, and his conception of self. In order to work effectively with ill and dying patients the nurse should have some understanding of where the patient is "coming from." Nurses should also understand their own philosophies and beliefs about illness, dying, and death. This sort of self-reflection is necessary if one is to understand diverse patients.

Illness, dying, and death all have an impact on the spiritual understandings of those undergoing these experiences. Illness can be a call to examine one's life and its spiritual meaning. Pre-death and near-death experiences involve major visionary events that may radically alter one's spiritual perspective. Medical practitioners who ignored these phenomena under the older scientific model have begun to accept and study these events. They also are acknowledging the validity of the patient's experience, at least to the extent of accepting the fact that the experience was real to the percipient.

## REFERENCES

Atwater, P. M. H. (1994). *Beyond the light: The mysteries and revelations of near-death experiences.* New York: Avon Books.

Barnum, B. (1996, Spring) The challenge of providing nursing care for the dying: An interview with Karen Soto, RN, BSN, and Rosalee Whyte, RN, BSN. *Nursing Leadership Forum.* 2(1), 34–37.

Berman, P. L. (1995). *The journey home.* New York: Pocket Books.

Brinkley, D., & Perry, P. (1994). *Saved by the light.* New York: Harper Paperbacks.

Da Avabhasa (1991). *Easy death* (2nd ed.). Clearlake, CA: Dawn Horse.

Kübler-Ross, E. (1969). *On death and dying.* New York: Macmillan.

Kübler-Ross, E. (1975). *Death: The final stage of growth.* Englewood Cliffs, NJ: Prentice Hall.

Longway, I. (1970, February/March). Toward a philosophy of nursing. *Journal of Adventist Education, 3,* 20–27.

Moody, R. A. (1975). *Life after life.* New York: Bantam Books.

Moody, R. A. (1977). *Reflections on life after life.* New York: Bantam Books.

Moody, R. A., & Perry, P. (1988). *The light beyond.* New York: Bantam Books.

Morse, M., & Perry, P. (1990). *Closer to the light.* New York: Random House.

Morse, M., & Perry, P. (1992). *Transformed by the light.* New York: Ballantine Books.

Morse, M., & Perry, P. (1993). *Reunions: Visionary encounters with departed loved ones.* New York: Ivy Books.

Newman, M. A. (2000). *Health as expanding consciousness* (2nd ed.). Boston: Jones and Bartlett.

Reverby, S. M. (1987). *Ordered to care: The dilemma of American nursing, 1850–1945.* Cambridge, England: Cambridge University Press.

Vash, C. L. (1994). *Personality and adversity: Psychospiritual aspects of rehabilitation.* New York: Springer.

Watson, J. (1999). *Nursing: Human science and human care: A theory of nursing.* Boston: Jones and Bartlett.

Weiss, B. L. (1992). *Many lives, many masters: Through time into healing.* New York: Simon & Schuster.

# PART IV

## Spirituality in Nursing's New Paradigm

$P$art IV deals with spirituality as it appears in nursing's adaptations of the new paradigm. Chapter 8 examines values and nursing theory components that may involve spirituality. The place of values in nursing theories is explored. Often nursing theories that claim to be based on humanitarian or spiritual values fail to present these elements as intrinsic parts of the given theories. Nursing has a long history of being value based, and values lie close to spirituality as we have defined it, for values arise from meaning.

Chapter 9 examines in detail some nursing theories fitting into the New Age paradigm, particularly comparing and contrasting the works of Dossey, Keegan, and Guzzetta (2000); Newman (2000); and Watson (1999), and finding some significant differences. These works, while not the only new paradigm nursing theories, typify the philosophies expressed and the positions taken.

This comparison illustrates the fact that not all theories dealing with spirituality take similar positions. Although no major new theorist has risen to expand on the themes of spirituality addressed in these three theories, the movement of holistic nursing practice has widely adopted and adapted these spiritually based theories.

Chapter 10 examines nursing and the concept of healing. This concept has importance in the present era in which nursing has been recognized as a healing art as much as a caring art. The difference between healing and curing will be examined under the lens of the new paradigm.

This chapter also examines one of the main boundary issues facing these new nursing theories: that of separating nursing from the domain claimed by the healing community, those healers who, while not nurses, function in much the same manner as some New Age nurses, often applying identical techniques. The boundary issue is critical: Are New Age nurse theorists really functioning as healers, not nurses? If they are different from healers, where does one draw the line between them?

Spirituality is a comfortable fit with the new paradigm, while it rubbed uncomfortably at of the edges of the older scientific paradigm. Indeed, the new paradigm has allowed nursing to return to its religious and spiritual roots, albeit in a radically changed form. Is spirituality here to stay in nursing theories? Or will it yield to the press of the medical orientation toward a scientific world-view?

# Chapter 8

## Spirituality as a Component in Nursing Theories

### THE PLACE OF VALUES IN NURSING THEORIES

Almost all nursing theories decree what the *good* nurse ought to do or be. Nursing theory is unique in this perspective. For example, in deriving a theory of chemistry, the chemist does not assert that hydrogen and oxygen *should* unite to make water, only that they do. Even the sociologist describes how people typically *do* act in any set of circumstances, not how they *ought* to act. True, social engineering can then attempt to create an environment where the preferred behaviors are most likely to occur, but the engineering occurs after the facts of behavior have been mapped.

Nurse theorists rarely start with how nurses *do* act. Instead, our theories tend to be prescriptive from the start, stating how nurses *should* act. Hence, valuing has been a part of nursing theory from the start.

Not all values are spiritual. Humanistic values exist apart from the search for a higher meaning or for a transcendent sense of self or God. Humanistic values of justice, liberty, equality, or service to mankind, for example, need not necessarily be based on a spiritual explanation that extends beyond the here and now.

Values often are used to tell us what makes the *good* nurse. Yet the term *good* has many meanings. In one connotation, *good* is a moral term related to one's value system, akin to rights and wrongs as well as duties and obligations, and the sources from which they flow. In another sense, *good* has a spiritual or religious connotation, meaning one is appropriately in tune with what is taken as God's will, universal harmony, or whatever spiritual conceptual viewpoint prevails. In yet another connotation, *good* is used in the way Aristotle talked about the good knife. In this sense of the word, *good* is applied when an object (or person) is effective in achieving desired goals. Hence, a good

107

knife is one that is sharp enough to cut. In this sense, *good* is moved out of the world of values into the world of effectiveness.

In nursing theories, we find a blend of these meanings, with some theorists applying one meaning, others blending several connotations. In some cases, one can determine the sense of good that is meant. Benner (1984; Benner, Tanner, & Chesla, 1996), for example, differentiates *excellent* exemplars (practice anecdotes already judged to be good) from those that are less good or deficient. Here the meaning is Aristotelian, that is, related to effectiveness.

Sometimes the link between a theory and its underlying value system is not as tight as the author might wish. Older theories often failed to integrate their value systems into their important theory components. A value system may lay like icing on a cake; that is, it could be scraped off without damaging the cake.

Values are better integrated into the New Age theories (see chapter 9) where the spiritual element is an intrinsic aspect of how the theory works. In older theories, it is not unusual to find a theorist proclaiming an ethical underpinning that is not intrinsic to the theory.

### THE COMPONENTS OF THEORY MODELS

Any comprehensive nursing theory has four components: content, process, context, and goal (Barnum, 1998). Where spirituality is an intrinsic part of a theory, it can comprise any one or several of these parts. If it is apart from these elements, it is a slogan rather than an essential part of the theory.

*Content* is the subject matter of a theory, the stable elements that are acted on or do the acting. *Process* is the method by which the theory works. It is the dynamic element, usually found in nursing acts or thoughts. *Goal* is the intended aim or objective of the theory, what one hopes to achieve. *Context* is the environment in which nursing occurs. It tells the nature of the world of nursing and the surroundings in which the patient exists (Barnum, 1998).

Spirituality often turns up as content, for example, in a theory where the human being is a composite of body, mind, and spirit. Another common use of spirit as content is in the form of a nursing diagnosis. This occurs in practice theories composed of nursing diagnoses, nursing outcomes, and nursing process. The various lists of nursing diagnoses are content items in these theories, although the particular diagnoses vary from list to list.

Spiritual diagnoses in these various theory formulations may involve any of the following: loss of faith, disturbance in one's value system, despair of receiving help from a spiritual source, or even hostility toward those suggesting spiritual assistance.

This common diagnosis-based nursing theory is a good one for learning how to differentiate content, process, goals, and context. In a sense this is easy to determine by the method of elimination. It is self-evident that "the nursing process" is a process element—actions to be taken. And the nursing outcomes lists clearly comprise the goal components of this theory.

By elimination, the nursing diagnoses must be content (stable subject matter). Although these diagnosis-based theories have no specified context, the various formulations come from a "scientific" ideology that may be said to comprise a partial context, in that—theoretically—anyone applying the theory to a given patient would arrive at the same diagnoses, same desired outcomes, and same suggested processes of care. The North American Nursing Diagnosis Association's (NANDA) (1999–2002) is one group whose list of diagnoses contains a spiritual component.

Process, as we said, represents the movement and action parts of a theory, whether the action is perceived as doing or thinking. A theory that has spirituality as process can be found in the early work of Longway (1970), who cited God as the source of man's power, power that could be cut off if a man fell out of the plan of redemption. Disease was a stoppage in man's power, and healing was the restoration of power by providing energy (the nurse's task, or one could say the "nursing process" of this theory).

> The method whereby energy is made available to man is by giving, motivated by love, for giving completes the circuit of God, the source of power. (p. 22)
>
> The aim of intervention is to supply energy to the individual, help him to lay hold of more energy for himself and thus to enable him to advance along the illness–wellness continuum as far as his limitations will permit. (p. 22)

The nursing process here is to complete a circuit of God and of power by supplying energy through love. This theory came about 20 years before the notion of energy transfer would become popular. The thoughts reflected by Longway are not that different from some of those developed in New Age theories of our time. They are an early forerunner of the now-common therapeutic touch.

Spiritual elements may also show up as theory goals or end points. Take, for example, Watson's (1999) theory. She explains man's end point this way:

> The person has one basic striving: to actualize the real self, thereby developing the spiritual essence of the self, and in the highest sense, to become more Godlike. In addition, each person seeks a sense of

harmony within the mind, body, and soul and thereby further inte-
grates, enhances, and actualizes the real self. The more one is able to
experience one's real self, the more harmony there will be within the
mind, body, and soul and a higher degree of health will exist. (p. 57)

Hence, in Watson's theory, we can identify a spiritual element as the end point
(actualizing the real self), the goal toward which each person strives.

Context is often the most difficult theory element to define. Although it
can loosely be called the environment, that environment may be physical, psychological, social, intellectual—whatever sort of environment provides the
background against which a theory is set. All the theories in chapter 9 take
place in an environment that can be said to be spiritual. Newman's context is
a world composed of expanding consciousness; Dossey's is the world of
transpersonal psychology (which extends beyond the personal into transpersonal realms of existence); and Watson's is a more traditional God-created
world with humans striving to be like God.

Spiritual elements may appear in the content, process, context, or goal
elements of a theory. This is not to say that spiritual elements may only appear
in one of these elements in a single theory. Indeed, in some of the New Age
theories, there are spiritual aspects to several elements.

## SUMMARY

Spiritual elements may appear in a theory as content, process, context, or goal.
Many nurses state a value system as background to their theories even where,
ironically, the value system is not an essential component of the theory itself.
Value systems may or may not include spiritual elements. Until recently, most
nursing theories had humanistic rather than spiritual value systems, but that
is changing.

## REFERENCES

Barnum, B. J. S. (1998). *Nursing theory: Analysis, application, evaluation* (5th ed.).
    Philadelphia: J. B. Lippincott.
Benner, P. (1984). *From novice to expert: Excellence and power in clinical nursing
    practices*. Menlo Park, CA: Addison-Wesley.
Benner, P., Tanner, C. A., & Chesla, C. A. (1996). *Expertise in nursing practice: Caring,
    clinical judgment, and ethics*. New York: Springer.
Dossey, B. M., Keegan, L., & Guzzetta, C. E. (Eds.). (3rd ed.). (2000). *Holistic nurs-
    ing: A handbook for practice* Gaithersburg, MD: Aspen.
Longway, I. (1970). Toward a philosophy of nursing. *Journal of Adventist Education,
    32*(3), 20–27.

Newman, M. A. (2000). *Health as expanding consciousness* (2nd ed.). Boston: Jones and Bartlett.

North American Nursing Diagnosis Association (1999–2002). *Nursing diagnoses: Definitions and classification*, 2001–2002 (4th ed.). Philadelphia: NurseCom.

Watson, J. (1999). *Nursing: Human science and human care: A theory of nursing.* Boston: Jones and Bartlett.

# Chapter 9

## Nursing Theorists in the New Paradigm

**A**ny time there is a basic change in the perception of what it means to be a human being, the goals and nature of nursing also undergo a change. So it has been in the newer nursing theories. In keeping with the emerging paradigm, many contemporary nursing theories contain some notion of the human being that involves continuous soul growth or expanding consciousness. Usually these concepts are goal-driven, with the person striving toward a higher good, God, or Source, however envisioned.

There is an early history in nursing of including spirit as part of the human being, then years of ignoring spirit, and now a resurgence of seeing spirit as subject matter for nursing. As we said in chapter 8, Longway (1970) was a theorist who made spirit central to her theory in an era when the scientific paradigm predominated. Working within a framework of holism, she defined a circuit of wholeness in which man had unlimited potential for growth and development, a wholeness denoting harmony among parts. To that notion she added the idea of God as the source of man's power—power that could be cut off if a man fell out of the plan of redemption. Longway described disease as a stoppage in man's power, and healing was the restoration of power by providing energy:

> The method whereby energy is made available to man is by giving, motivated by love, for giving completes the circuit of God, the source of power. (p. 22)
>
> The aim of intervention is to supply energy to the individual, help him to lay hold of more energy for himself and thus to enable him to advance along the illness–wellness continuum as far as his limitations will permit. (p. 22)

This description comes close to some of the theories in the new paradigm. Because Longway's nurse heals by supplying energy, the theory is one in which the nurse is a healer as well as a caretaker. Published over thirty years ago, Longway's theory did not start a spiritual resurgence. That had to wait until the emergence of a new world paradigm.

Ironically, her work sounds like contemporary nursing theories of therapeutic touch and energy movement. Typically, these newer formulations attempt to tie these energy processes to contemporary physics. As Slater (1995), a nurse, says:

> The author [Slater] contends that all EH [energetic healing] methods are variations of one theme: the ability to consciously regulate what physicists call quantum and EM [electromagnetic] energy. (p. 209)

Brennan (1987), a non-nurse healer, gives a similar explanation:

> Through experiments in the past few decades, physicists found matter to be completely mutable, and on the subatomic level, matter does not exist with certainty in definite places, but rather shows "tendencies" to exist. All particles can be transmuted into other particles. They can be created from energy and can vanish into energy. (p. 24)
>
> I suggest that since we are inseparable parts of that whole, we can enter into a holistic state of being, become the whole, and tap into the creative powers of the universe to instantaneously heal anyone anywhere. (p. 28)

This shift from Longway's God to modern physics did not mark an end of the "spiritual connection" so much as an attempt to arrive at a "theory of everything." The attempt was (and still is) to tie together the human being, God, and physics. Energy and its movement, then, was seen as linking all three of these subjects. Linking the human being and God led to a new psychology, that of transpersonal development. As we indicated in chapter 4, transpersonal psychologists identify various levels of development beyond self-actualization, most of which would meet our definition of spiritual (see Wilber, 1980).

Newman (1999) noted the need for continual development in the human being:

> People who strive to maintain stability in their lives by shielding themselves from interactions that might disturb their equilibrium do not appear to move ahead to higher states of consciousness. (p. 229)
>
> We evolve by having our equilibrium thrown off balance, then discovering how to attain a new temporary state of balance, and moving on to another phase of disequilibrium. (p. 229)

Such continuous progressing brings one to the spiritual stages of being proposed in transpersonal psychology. One can see a practice problem in the making here: Can a less spiritually developed nurse (suppose a very young nurse) help a more spiritually developed patient? Spirituality, seen from a developmental perspective, raises questions as to the nurse's qualifications. Unlike psychological and sociological aspects of nursing, spiritual maturity isn't achieved by learning alone. If "body work" is the primary role, the level of the nurse's spiritual maturity isn't critical, but if spiritual assistance is part of the role, there is a potential problem.

(Throughout this chapter, the term *body work* is used to signal those aspects of care that require the most intensive levels of technology, for example, treatments, medications, and other "things to be done." We realize that for most new paradigm theories there is no absolute divide between these forms of care for the person and care for other components of the human being, such as mind and spirit. However, we'll use the term *body work* to indicate the most hands-on elements of nursing care.)

## COMPARISON OF THREE SPIRITUAL NURSING THEORIES

Three nurse theorists with spiritually based theories have attained prominence in nursing. In varying degrees, they diverge from traditional spiritual formulations toward New Age theories of spirituality. We'll look at Watson, Dossey and colleagues, and Newman in the order of their distance from traditional Judeo-Christian patterns of religion. Figure 9.1 provides the reader with a brief review of their theories. If the reader is not familiar with these theories, he should refer to their books listed in the Reference section of this chapter.

### Theory Elements

As was stated in chapter 8, theories can be parsed into elements of content, process, goal, and context. Diagramming a theory (as in Figure 9.1) is useful in revealing its differences from (or similarities to) other theories.

In looking at Watson's (1999) theory, for example, we find: *content* as human soul comprised of body-mind-spirit; *process* as interpersonal caring; *goal* as harmony among parts; and *context* as a spiritual God-ordered world. Looked at in this way, at least three of Watson's components have spiritual elements. Notice the soul has replaced the scientific paradigm's bio-psycho-social human; he is now comprised of body, mind, and *spirit*. As Watson (1999) says:

| THEORIST | Watson | Dossey and Colleagues | Newman |
|----------|--------|------------------------|--------|
| CONTENT | Human soul (Body-mind-spirit) | Bio-psycho-social-spiritual person | Evolving consciousness |
| PROCESS | Interpersonal caring | Doing/Being | Repatterning |
| GOAL(S) | Harmony of body-mind-spirit Striving to be like God | Healing/evolving of transpersonal self | Continuous evolution of self as mind |
| CONTEXT | Spiritual God-ordered world | Transcendent reality mediated by mind, neuro-psycho-immunology | World as mental and evolving |
| DISEASE | Disharmony among parts | Obstruction in evolution toward next life phase | Signal of a need for change, ready for higher evolution |
| HEALTH | Harmony of parts | Personal growth, move toward transpersonal | Continuous by expanding the consciousness |
| GOD | The Source man strives to emulate The Creator | The ground of being to which man is similar/identical | Evolving consciousness of which man is a part |

**FIGURE 9.1** Comparison of three spiritual nursing theories.

The concept of the soul, as used here refers to the *geist*, spirit, inner self, or essence of the person, which is tied to a greater sense of self-awareness, a higher degree of consciousness, an inner strength, and a power that can expand human capacities and allow a person to transcend his or her usual self. The higher sense of consciousness and valuing of inner self can cultivate a fuller access to the intuitive and even sometimes allow uncanny, mystical, or miraculous experiences, modes of thought, feelings, and actions that we have all experienced at some points in our life, but from which our rational, scientific cultures bar us. (p. 46)

Each of the assumptions underlying the view of human life is that each of us is a magnificent spiritual being who has often been undernourished and reduced to a physical, materialistic being. We know both rationally and intuitively, however, that a person's human predicament may not be related to the external, physical world as much as to the person's inner world as lived and experienced. Awareness of oneself as a spiritual being opens up infinite possibilities. (p. 46)

Watson focuses on the theory-building facet of incorporating spirituality into nursing practice:

The notion of a human soul is nothing new or original. It is, however, unusual to include it in a theory. The closest concept in psychology and nursing are concepts like self, inner self, "I," me, self-actualization, and so on. The bold attempt to acknowledge and try to incorporate a concept of the soul in a nursing theory is a reflection of an alternative position that nursing is now free to take. The new concept breaks from the traditional medical science model and is also a reflection of the scientific times. The evolution of the history and philosophy of science now allows some attention to metaphysical views that would have been unacceptable at an earlier point in time. (p. 49)

Watson's theory of spirit emerged from an earlier theory of caring. It is not unusual for spirituality to become more significant as a theorist ages. Watson (1999) says:

The world of the spirit and soul becomes increasingly more important as a person grows and matures as an individual and as humankind evolves collectively. (p. 56)

The person has one basic striving: to actualize the real self, thereby developing the spiritual essence of the self, and in the highest sense, to become more Godlike. (p. 57)

These thoughts push the envelope of traditional religion by indicating that the human can and should transcend self, and seek mystic and miraculous experiences.

In looking at Dossey, Keegan, and Guzzetta's (2000) theory, we find: *content* as bio-psycho-social-spiritual human; *process* as doing/being; *goal* as healing/evolving of the transpersonal self; and *context* as a transcendent reality mediated by mind using neuro-psycho-immunology systems.

Dossey and Guzzetta (Dossey, Keegan, & Guzzetta, 2000) work to integrate these elements of the human (bio-psycho-social-spiritual). They make a point that the spiritual is as important as the other elements:

> [e]ach component of the bio-psycho-social-spiritual model is interdependent and interrelated. It is necessary to address all these components to achieve optimal therapeutic results. (p. 9)

Using the third edition of their book (Dossey, Keegan, & Guzzetta, 2000), it is difficult to specify with certainty the elements of this theory because so many new authors have been added, each contributing a special twist. Yet general themes are consistent and in agreement with the second edition, which had more depth on philosophic issues and no contributors outside of the four authors (Dossey, Keegan, Guzzetta, & Kolkmeier, 1995). I am assuming that the principles not detailed in the new edition are still underlying assumptions of the third edition. Indeed, the presented material is consistent with the same viewpoints, even where philosophic underpinnings have been omitted from the text.

In the new edition, Burkhardt and Jacobson (2000) further define the elements of spirituality as (1) connectedness with the Absolute, (2) connectedness with nature, (3) connectedness with others, and (4) connectedness with self.

The nursing process is very important to Dossey and colleagues. Dossey and Guzzetta (Dossey, Keegan, & Guzzetta, 2000) specify these two techniques:

> Doing therapies include almost all forms of modern medicine, such as medications, procedures, dietary manipulations, radiation, and acupuncture. In contrast, being therapies do not employ things but utilize states of consciousness, such as imagery, prayer, meditation, and quiet contemplation, as well as the presence and intention of the nurse. These techniques are therapeutic because of the power of the psyche to affect the body. (p. 12)

Further, they differentiate the source of these different methods as falling on two ends of a healing spectrum: rational or paradoxical:

> "Doing" therapies fall into the rational healing category, because they make sense to our linear, intellectual thought processes. . . On the other hand, "being" therapies fall into the paradoxical healing category, because they frequently happen without a scientific explanation. (p. 13)

Paradoxical therapies include, among others, biofeedback, placebos, miracle cures, prayer, and faith. This division of the nurse's role into doing and being allows for an addition of new techniques to older therapies without negating the older ones. The additional element of spirit has been neatly integrated into the content element of theory as one component of the human as well as the nursing process.

Several major shifts have taken place here away from Watson's position. First, where Watson's human strived to be like God, Dossey and colleagues say man is similar or identical to God—Divine reality in their terms (Dossey, Keegan, Guzzetta, Kolkmeier, 1995). With some tentativeness, they assert at least the possibility that the human being is part of God, not separate.

Second, their process is rather clever in that they don't deny the necessity for "body work" (doing); they simply add a new component, being, and the effects that can be achieved by presence in a meaningful way. They also add new types of doing that reflect and work with newer perceptions of the human being, such as energetic healing. In essence, they can add a whole new group of therapies without doing away with that peritoneal dialysis. This approach is less limiting than Watson's reliance on interpersonal caring.

Third, Dossey and colleagues have tried to put whatever components of the new paradigm lend themselves to such treatment into the scientific research model (e.g., the neuro-psycho-immunology work). Yet they do not bind themselves to the scientific method, calling many *being* effects paradoxical.

As with Watson's theory, the theory of Dossey and colleagues is vastly spiritual. One could argue that all four of their theory components have spiritual elements.

Newman's theory shows the most extreme deviance from the traditional religious viewpoint. Looking briefly at Newman's theory we find *content* as mind/evolving consciousness; *process* as repatterning; *goal* as continuous evolution of self as mind; and *context* as a world that is mental and evolving. Viewed this way, Newman's theory has spiritual elements in at least three components.

The content, mind/consciousness, is ever evolving, one might say, toward God, albeit not the usual omniscient and omnipotent God but one that is continually growing and developing. Indeed, expanding consciousness becomes equated with God. It is the human being striving to be all he can as a component of that changing God. He can't help but participate in God because all consciousness—from inanimate objects to spiritual beings beyond the human level—participate in God:

There is openness of interaction throughout the entire spectrum of consciousness. The human being interacts with animals and plants on one end of the spectrum and astral and spiritual beings at the other end. All creation is in constant and instantaneous contact. (Newman, 2000, p. 35)

[l]ife is evolving in the direction of higher levels of consciousness; that complementary forces of order and disorder maintain a fluctuating field that periodically transcends itself and shifts into a higher order of functioning; and that in humans this evolutionary process is facilitated by insight and involves a transcendence of the spatial-temporal self to a spiritual realm. (p. 43)

Newman's God is not some personal all-knowing being but comes closer to an intelligent energy, a pattern seeking further evolution and knowledge of itself.

Thus, each of our sample New Age theories has some concept of the human being's place in relation to spirit/God. Despite their great differences, each theorist accepts some version of the new paradigm and has spiritual elements inherent in the nursing theories rather than present as a mere overlay.

### The Self

Diagramming each theory allows for an easy comparison of specific topics. For example, in relation to the *self*, one might make these observations. Watson envisions a developing unique self, (not a part of God, although perhaps a "child" of God), while Dossey and colleagues claim a self who may be similar or identical to God. Newman describes a self definitely merging with, or becoming aware of its participation in, the larger whole that constitutes her notion of God. In all three cases, the person is conceived as entering yet another developmental phase beyond rational maturity, beyond Maslow's self-actualization, into a transpersonal level of being or to some level of participation in a consciousness we can legitimately label as spiritual.

All of these authors mention transpersonal development. Dossey and colleagues and Newman closely follow the work of transpersonal psychologists. Watson gives fewer details concerning her ideas of the transpersonal, so it may or may not involve transpersonal psychology. In relation to transpersonal development, one might cite Wilber (1980), who sees the reemergence of a spiritual/religious state (transpersonal) not as a return to primitive religion but as the next step in evolution beyond the limitations of the rational phase of human development.

## Disease

It is also interesting to compare these theorists on their ideas of *disease*. For Watson and Dossey and colleagues, disease is mostly negative, that is disharmony and obstruction respectively. The patient and the nurse work to get rid of disease. These views contrast with Newman's in which disease may be therapeutic, a shock that allows the person to reorganize in his struggle toward a new level of harmony (new patterning).

Newman's conception is reminiscent of Levinson's (1977) work in which he saw developmental stages as static planes between transitional periods of upheaval. For Newman, then, one might postulate illness to be a natural part of the pattern: the upheaval that signals an opportunity to repattern at a higher level. As she says:

It seems strange to say . . . but disease may be the way a person gets in touch with his or her pattern. Many of us have lived our lives in such a way that we have not become fully aware of our selves or our own pattern. The pattern may then manifest itself in a more "unconscious" manner, in terms of changes that may be interpreted as maladaptive, or disease, but which may represent movement to a higher level of consciousness. (Newman, 2000, p. 20)

This does not mean that Newman would expect the disease to remain, but that it would recede when the lesson it brought was heeded.

## The Nursing Process

Theorists also differ on just what the nurse does with the patient, and, equally important, how she fulfills (or fails to fulfill) the expected nursing duties. In our three illustrative theories, we see a cascade of development in which the nurse's justification for body work is uncomplicated, tenuous, or very difficult.

Dossey and colleagues have the easiest time of it because their model, even though it is radically different, is the closest to a traditional model in the element of caregiving. Their being/doing process allows easily for physical care. They have not dismissed the traditional elements of man so much as added to them. Their patient is a bio-psycho-social-spiritual entity. A new element has been added to the old mix without canceling out the old.

Watson's (1999) nurse justifies her process, but the rationale is harder to come by. Because disease is disharmony for Watson's nurse, it is her job to help restore the patient's harmony. Caring is the chief vehicle that the nurse uses to restore harmony:

The actual concrete action of caring can transcend the value (and pass it on). Embedded in this idea is the notion that caring values and actions can be contagious, at an individual and systemic level, if sufficient conditions are met. The value of caring is grounded in the self-transcending creative nurse. (p. 32)

Watson blends meanings of caring in the emotive sense of "feeling for" and in the sense of "taking care of." Yet her focus is on the emotive link. Indeed, Watson discusses with great dismay the modern technology as a monster that has swallowed up the caring element of nursing. Clearly this refers to the emotive aspect of caring, not the act of physical taking care of. Care of the body is justified, however, because the body is an access point to the person:

A nurse may have access to a person's mind, emotions, and inner self indirectly through any sphere—mind, body or soul—provided the physical body is not perceived or treated as separate from the mind and emotions and higher sense of self (soul). (p. 50)

Watson, therefore, justifies physical acts of care as vehicles to reach the nonphysical parts of man (the important parts in her theory). Her nurse is motivated to do this because the illness is a symptom of a disharmony of the soul; it is a signal that the parts need a positive change. She defines the human as body, mind, and spirit, so that gives her permission to tend to body and mind as well as spirit. Unlike Dossey and colleagues, however, Watson appears to give a heavier focus to the spiritual element.

Newman's theory of health as expanding consciousness creates great difficulties in justification of the nurse's care of the body, especially because Newman says that disease and wellness are all simply parts of the process of consciousness expansion. Newman warns against disrupting what may be a clarion call to a needed change. In other words, the disease may be a teacher and, as such, should not be countervailed in a manner that masks its meaning.

How or why, then, does the nurse help in this journey of consciousness expanding and evolving? One can argue that she helps the patient interpret the message of the disease; she helps the patient understand his pattern. Changing the pattern will likely remove the disease; it will no longer be needed as a teacher. Of course, in seeing the disease as something to be overcome, we have somewhat stepped outside of Newman's notion that disease and wellness are equal parts of the consciousness-evolving process.

Helping the patient discover and change the pattern constitutes justifiable nursing behavior in this nursing model. However, we must ask if this activity can justify such acts as giving the injection or changing the dialysis fluid.

Often modern medicine acts to remove the disease with little interest in why it arose in the first place. There is a sense in Newman's model that nursing and medicine work at odds, medicine aiming to relieve the disease while the nurse struggles to make it meaningful for the patient before the physician succeeds. And, of course, the nurse—if hired by a hospital, for example—is expected to participate in the removal of the teacher (the disease).

Because of this mechanism and the fact that her goal has nothing to do with the body, except as a learning environment, Newman's model has the greatest difficulty among our three sample theories in justifying basic normative nursing care, that is, tending to the body, participating in the body cure plan. Perhaps for this reason, her book is full of illustrations of care. Still, Newman (2000) has the most difficult rationalization for body work. She assumes that if the patient evolves, his disease will be affected positively.

Hence all of our theorists can account for physical care of the patient, albeit in a tenuous way for some, more directly for others. Obviously, these new ideologies have impact on nursing practice. The nurse who sees illness as a human opportunity to rise to a new level of existence (Newman and Dossey) will treat the patient differently than the nurse who sees it as disharmony of the soul, and all of these nurses will respond differently than the nurse who sees illness as an impersonal accident of fate.

A major question remains as to what specifically nurses will *do* with the spiritual aspect of nursing where it is included, and how they qualify for the work involved.

While Watson's (1999) work describing spirituality moves beyond the older paradigm theories, her work on therapeutics is less revolutionary. Her prescription, establishing a transpersonal caring relationship, sounds much like the existential theories of earlier ages:

A transpersonal caring relationship connotes a special kind of human care relationship—a union with another person—high regard for the whole person and their being-in-the-world. Caring, in this sense, is viewed as the moral ideal of nursing where there is the utmost concern for human dignity and preservation of humanity. Human care can begin when the nurse enters into the life space or phenomenal field of another person, is able to detect the other person's condition of being (spirit, soul), feels this condition within him- or herself, and responds to the condition in such a way that the recipient has a release of subjective feelings and thoughts he or she had been longing to release. As such, there is an intersubjective flow between the nurse and patient. (p. 63)

This process seems, perhaps, to require less "spiritual preparation" and more psychological preparation than the other theories, more human sensitivity and interpersonal skills. This process does not deal specifically with spirit. For example, the same process would assist mind, especially the emotive state.

In contrast, Dossey and Guzzetta (2000) add something more specific to one's spiritual status when they write of being skills:

> In contrast, being therapies do not employ things but use states of consciousness, such as imagery, prayer, meditation, and quiet contemplation, as well as the presence and intention of the nurse. (p. 12)

Hence, in this theory there is more direct spiritual technology (to be discussed in chapter 11).

Newman's explanation is more metaphysical, perhaps less directive. She relates the nurse to the client's rhythm of transition, with the two people relating in a paradigm of wholeness:

> The nature of nursing is found in the nurse's relationship with the client, a relationship characterized by a rhythmic coming together and moving apart as clients encounter disruption of their organized, predictable state and moving through disorganization and unpredictability to a higher, organized state. (Newman, 1999, p. 228)

### Value and Task Clashes

From these sample New Age theories of nursing, we begin to see that the New Age theorist faces a peculiar problem, that is, that patients and nurses may have radically different expectations. Patients expect that nurses will take care of them when they are ill. Most patients hope that nurses will be caring concerning their emotional needs but expect that nurses will take care of their physical needs, whether the care be hygienic, medicinal, or performance of treatments.

If a nurse were introduced to the patient as a professional who is there to expand his consciousness or put his soul back in harmony, many patients might be confused. This is not what they expect. Why, then, are nurses allowed to fill such roles (when and where they do so)? Primarily because, at the same time, they tend to the patient's body.

A theory problem arises when one asserts that a nurse from these paradigms must understand high technology as well as philosophy of the soul. Whether nurses like it or not, most institutions hire them to perform acts unrelated to the soul, and they are expected to perform those technical acts with skill and knowledge. If the nurse fails to understand the dynamics of peritoneal dialysis, for example, she is a hazard. And few institutions will hire her "merely" to tend to the patient's evolving consciousness or to establish harmony.

Pragmatically, most nursing takes place when someone is ill. If nursing is care of the soul, then a person who identifies a soul (spiritual) deficiency might need a nurse even if his body is healthy. This is not to denigrate these New Age theories of nursing, but simply to point out that they may be at odds with the goals and functions of most institutions that employ nurses. Some nurses have suggested that the cure for this problem is for nurses to work elsewhere other than in ill care. This brings us back to the question raised earlier of whether these New Age philosophies of nursing are really about nursing or about some new profession in the making.

Can alternate philosophies survive in the same institution? Or will nursing depart from the ideologies that still dominate in most of our health care institutions? Will nurses set up their own institutions based on a different set of values? The issue is perhaps reminiscent of the cultural complexities that arise in those developing countries where modern medicine exists side by side with the shaman and folk medicine. The alternate systems (New Age theories and the medical model) may exist side by side, but they share little philosophic common ground as typically formulated.

Can the two elements (body care and soul care) be done simultaneously? Of course. Can a theory rationalize why the two elements are irrevocably joined? That is more difficult. Worse, must the nurse do what she perceives as her true work (soul work) under the guise of doing something else (body work)?

It is true that the New Age theorists have a place for the body, but the truth is that the body is not paramount. Dossey and colleagues, we have noted, escape this problem somewhat with their theory of doing and being. But for other new paradigm theories, one must ask: Is the practice of the New Age nurse deceptive? Does the patient's weakened condition simply make him a target of opportunity? If New Age nursing is care of the soul, is it usurping the field of those perceived to be more prepared for that task, namely priests, ministers, rabbis, and other religious leaders? What if the patient prefers to select his own spiritual advisor?

Indeed, we must pose several questions concerning this new addition to nursing's role: Should nurses be in the spirit business? If not, to whom do we pass the baton? If we are in the spiritual business, what are we to do about the fact that both patients and nurses may come from different paradigms, let alone different religious beliefs and different levels of spiritual maturity?

Nursing theories in the new paradigm, however cast, move nursing into strange new territory: care and fostering of the soul or spirit. This is an arena in which nursing prescriptions are beginning and are often subsumed under other holistic practices.

Although there are differences among the nurse theorists—with Dossey and colleagues and Newman perhaps closer to each other than to Watson—taken together, they represent a new direction. They accept a radically revised view of the human being and his place in the cosmos.

This is not to say that a reconciliation is not possible between body work and soul work. . Wilber (1996) proposes a comprehensive reality model that can subsume the scientific model within a larger framework, allowing for other domains, other processes; that is, this model could include both the scientific paradigm and the New Age paradigm without internal contradiction. Among other differentiations, his model contains divisions between interior and exterior phenomena:

> But notice that these are all *exterior* descriptions—it's what these holons look like from the outside, in an objective and empirical manner. Thus, in a scientific text, you will find the limbic system, for example, described in detail—its components, its biochemistry, when and how it evolved, how it relates to other parts of the organism, and so on. And you will probably find it mentioned that the limbic system is the home of certain very fundamental *emotions*, certain basic types of sex and aggression and fear and desire, whether that limbic system appears in horses or humans or apes.
>
> But of those emotions, of course, you will not find much description, because emotions pertain to the interior experience of the limbic system. These emotions and the awareness that goes with them are what the holon with a limbic system *experiences from within*, on the *inside*, in its *interior*. And *objective* scientific descriptions are not much interested in that interior consciousness, because that interior space cannot be accessed in an objective, empirical fashion. (pp. 75–76)

Hence, Wilber's model allows for diverse kinds of phenomena, each studied by its own appropriate methods. Internal and external phenomena exist as two viewpoints, each with its own domains of inquiry, research, and practice.

By having a theory large enough to contain both viewpoints, a resolution between scientific and New Age paradigms is possible. The phenomena of the new paradigm obviously cannot be subsumed under the scientific model. Nor can all New Age phenomena be subjected to the scientific method of the external view. But the scientific model and the New Age paradigm can be subsumed in a theory large enough to contain both of them.

Nursing has not yet developed a theory that adequately permits this reconciliation. At present new paradigm theories vie for preeminence with theories based on a scientific model. In actual nursing programs of education, schools tend to adopt a holistic approach or a scientific model rather than a synthesis of both. At present, the two philosophies, with their associated methods, have little tolerance for each other. Some schools with a holistic, new paradigm curriculum flaunt the fact that their students learn little of modern care techniques. And schools with a scientific model tend to dismiss all new paradigm proposals as hokum. A goal for the future is to create a theory that incorporates both elements without stigmatizing either.

## NEW AGE AND SPIRITUALITY: ARE THEY THE SAME?

The question of whether a theory is spiritual is critical for the purposes of this book. The answer depends on the meaning of spirit. Is expanded consciousness, for example, merely a refinement on accidental man, a protoplasmic blip in a universe that is itself a chance occurrence? Or is the whole process of human development a movement from or toward some teleological meaning? Do all levels of supraconscious perception involve spirituality? Or can they be conceptualized scientifically, from some human potential framework?

Similarly, does the spiritual always involve some concept of God or a higher power? What if the images of that higher power are as diverse as that of "Big Daddy in the Sky" and an abstract set of principles or energy? What is it that makes something spiritual? One can envision cases where a New Age theorist might feel that a rigidly formalized religion had lost its original spiritual zest.

The opposite case certainly applies: a fundamentalist might find nothing spiritual and a lot sinful about new paradigm beliefs. The issue is the old one: If one holds a given perspective as the only valid spiritual starting point, then everything that doesn't start from that premise is judged not to be spiritual.

Recall that in this book we have defined spirituality as meaning a person's search for, or expression of, his connection to a greater and meaningful context. For some people, that connection will be seen as a connection with God; for others it may be finding their place in the universe, and that may involve in-depth searching for a greater sense of self.

## SUMMARY

Most new paradigm theories of nursing deal with interesting, emerging content such as transpersonal psychology, aspects of transition and temporality, concepts of self-growth as cure, and changing notions of God, physics, and the human being's place in the greater reality. Spirituality plays a stronger part in these newer nursing theories than was the case in theories arising when nursing was striving to prove itself "scientific." Spiritual aspects of New Age theories show up in all the elements: content, process, goals, and context, often in several aspects within a single theory.

Within a New Age ideology, there is space for wide diversity in nursing theories, as has been illustrated here by theories of Watson, Dossey and colleagues, and Newman. Most, but not all, New Age theories associate human development (however described) with man striving for God. These new interpretations of man as essentially spirit instead of primarily bio-psycho-social, have had, and will continue to have, major impact on how nursing is perceived.

## REFERENCES

Brennan, B. A. (1987). *Hands of light: A guide to healing through the human energy field*. New York: Bantam Books.

Burkhardt, M. A., & Jacobson, M. G. N. (2000). Spirituality and health. In B. M. Dossey, L. Keegan, & C. E. Guzzetta (Eds.), *Holistic nursing: A handbook for practice* (3rd ed., pp. 91–121). Gaithersburg, MD: Aspen.

Dossey, B. M., & Guzzetta, C. E. (2000). Holistic nursing practice. In B. M. Dossey, L. Keegan, & C. E. Guzzetta (Eds.), *Holistic nursing: A handbook for practice* (3rd ed., pp. 5–33). Gaithersburg, MD: Aspen.

Dossey, B. M., Keegan, L., & Guzzetta, C. E. (Eds.). (2000). *Holistic nursing: A handbook for practice* (3rd ed.). Gaithersburg, MD: Aspen.

Dossey, B. M., Keegan, L., Guzzetta, C. E., & Kolkmeier, L. G. (Eds.). (1995). *Holistic nursing: A handbook for practice* (2nd ed.). Gaithersburg, MD: Aspen.

Levinson, D. J. (1977). The mid-life transition: A period in adult psychological development. *Psychiatry, 2*(40), 99–112.

Longway, I. (1970). Toward a philosophy of nursing. *Journal of Adventist Education, 32*(3), 20–27.

Newman, M. A. (1999). The rhythm of relating in a paradigm of wholeness. *Image: Journal of Nursing Scholarship, 31*(3), 227–230.

Newman, M. A. (2000). *Health as expanding consciousness* (2nd ed.). Boston: Jones and Bartlett.

Slater, V. E. (1995, September). Toward an understanding of energetic healing, Part 1. *Journal of Holistic Nursing, 13*(3), 209–224.

Watson, J. (1999). *Nursing: Human science and human care: A theory of nursing*. Boston: Jones and Bartlett.

Wilber, K. (1980). *The Atman project*. Wheaton, IL: Quest Books.

Wilber, K. (1996). *A brief history of everything*. Boston: Shambhala.

# Chapter 10

## Nursing and Healing

### HEALING VERSUS CURING

At one time, the dichotomy in health care was between *caring* and *curing*, with nursing doing the caring and medicine performing the curing. That dichotomy was dissolved forever when nurse practitioners moved into primary practice: nurses then definitively cared *and* cured. The next dichotomy to arise was between *curing* and *healing*. Simply put, people speak of curing a disease and healing a person. Hence curing is a term used most often in the scientific paradigm, while healing is used more often in the new paradigm and certainly in relationship to spirituality.

Many theorists consider curing a small subset of healing. Dossey, Keegan, Guzzetta, and Kolkmeier (1995) differentiate between curing and healing in this way:

> Healing is not just the curing of symptoms. It is the exquisite blending of technology with caring, love, compassion, and creativity. Healing is a lifelong journey into understanding the wholeness of human existence. . . . Healing is learning to open what has been closed so that we can expand our inner potentials. . . . A nurse healer is one who facilitates another person's growth toward wholeness (body-mind-spirit) or who assists another in the recovery from illness or in the transition to peaceful death. (p. xxvi)

Quinn (2000) reflects a similar viewpoint:

> Although curing follows a usual or predictable path, healing is always creative and unpredictable in both process and outcome. In textbooks

on curing, the events that will be probably parts of recovery and the time line are described, and the actual progress of the patient is measured against these referents. (p. 42)

Healing as a process of emergence does not lend itself to the type of outcome measurement usually applied to curing. It is one thing to evaluate whether the signs and symptoms of disease are still present. It is quite another to determine if there has been a shift at any level of this person's body-mind-spirit. (p. 42)

A similar difference between healing and curing is made by McGlone (1990), who says that healing means to be made whole and involves an awakening of a deeper sense of self. In these descriptions, as is the case in many New Age nursing theories, healing has more to do with person than with disease. Indeed, the person might be judged to have "healed" even though an illness remains. For purposes of this chapter, we'll use the term that deals with the whole person, that is, *healing*.

The term *healer* is even more difficult to define than healing. At one time, the word was associated with the religious healer who worked miracles in one dramatic gesture, with the person being healed instantly, or, as was usually the case, cured.

Today, few healers bring about dramatic instant miracle cures. Most treat their clients over a period of time. Further, although nurses make up a large number of today's healers, they don't own the turf. There are many other health professionals who are healers, as well as healers who entirely lack medical credentials.

## HEALING MODALITIES

One can contrast healing in the new paradigm and healing in traditional religion. As we'll see in chapters 11 and 12, the methods in these two orientations may be somewhat similar, with only the interpretations of what is happening as different. We'll look briefly at both cases.

### New Paradigm Healing

The new paradigm healer's efforts call for a new definition of the human being. People who work as New Age healers usually see the human being as having the following characteristics.

1. A person's thoughts have greater impact on his/her body than was conceptualized in older paradigms. Techniques such as guided imagery may be used for healing because they can reprogram the body as well

as the mind. A person's thoughts, in some new paradigm models, are part of an evolving God.

2. The body stores emotions and events in various body parts, and these emotions may be affected through forms of body work such as massage, rolfing, and reflexology.

3. The human being extends beyond the visible tactile body to include different layers of an etheric body (aura) that begins where one's skin leaves off. Layers of the aura also are associated with the various energy centers (chakras) that are proposed to govern the body. The energy layers of the aura have different vibratory frequencies and properties and may give evidence of disease before the body changes become apparent. The aura may be manipulated by a knowledgeable healer.

4. Personal energy and/or a universal energy exist and may be tapped for healing. Systems of energy movement usually involve regulating energy through the hands (e.g., in therapeutic touch, reiki, and other methods).

5. The human body and the perceived reality are influenced by the state of consciousness. Levels and types of awareness in both the healer and the client may be manipulated to produce changes.

6. The human is an integral part of the earth and, by extension, of the universe.

These same assumptions underlie not only healing, but many of the new paradigm therapies discussed in chapter 11. Further, these proposals, which might have sounded frivolous at one time, draw substance from many sources, from modern physics, to a growing influx of Eastern philosophies, to the successes of practitioners using such a belief structure. Nevertheless, acceptance of these beliefs is far from universal. Many physicians, for example, have great difficulty believing in a system describing components that cannot be identified on dissection (chakra energy vortices, for example).

Many forms of healing employ these principles, including such approaches as energetic healing, sound therapy, rolfing, shamanic practice, neurofeedback, thought field therapy, aroma therapy, essential oil therapy, and many others. The growth of complementary medicine, starting perhaps with herbology, gives evidence to the growing interest in the new paradigm views and prescriptions. Even when people do not understand the notions of the human being with which the healer works, they often are glad for the effects of the therapy.

### Bioenergetic Healing

Energetic (otherwise termed *energic*) healing, movement of energy with the hands, is perhaps the most common new paradigm healing technique. Brennan

(1993), a non-nurse healer, says that we all use movement of energy, whether or not we realize it:

> How you are in any given moment is expressed through your energy. When you learn to regulate your moods and therefore the nature of your energy and your energy flow, you will soon be using your energy for healing. This is what healers do. They simply learn to perceive and regulate their energy in order to utilize it for healing. (p. 3)

Laurie and Tucker (1993), also non-nurses, give more details about the dangers of misusing energies:

> But caution must be exercised for it is possible by will and desire to transmit one's energy and leave oneself depleted. This happens when the healer doesn't understand the process. Energy can be gathered from all forms of life, not just other humans. (p. 145)

In their work, these authors describe how a healer can draw energy from other sources, becoming a channel rather than draining one's own energy. Authors of various works on energy tell the practitioner to draw the external energy from various sources: the atmosphere, the molten core of the earth, the heavens. Drawing on external energy, then, seems to be an act of active imagination, the act being more important than the envisioned source. Use of imagination for various healing purposes will be discussed later in this chapter.

Quinn (1994), a nurse healer, says much the same thing about acquiring energy when explaining the nursing procedure of therapeutic touch. She indicates that care and love are cosmic forces that comprise universal energy:

> The nurse in a centered state of consciousness accesses this energy and it becomes available to him or her as well as to the patient. (p. 67)

Dossey (1995) defines the nurse healer in relation to energy flow:

> The healer is like a channel, passively yet, paradoxically, with discernment permitting the cosmic energy to flow unobstructedly through his or her own energy fields into those of the client. The healer must be aware of the disturbances in the client's wholeness at high levels . . . like an electrical transformer, the healer transforms the prodigious cosmic energy into a form that can be used by the client's body-mind-spirit system. (p. 43)

Unlike some approaches to medicine, in the new paradigm, the patient is active in healing endeavors.

Quinn (1989) describes that patient's part in the healing. She sees the healer as midwife to an internal healing process in the patient:

> Healing is a total, organismic, synergistic *response* that must emerge from within the individual if recovery and growth are to be accomplished. . . . The Haelan Effect is the activation of the innate, diverse, synergistic, and multidimensional self-healing mechanism which manifests as emergence and repatterning of relationship. (p. 554)

Schwartz (2002), a psychologist healer who uses thought field therapy, also believes that the patient's part in healing is essential:

> All healing is actually self-healing, a journey of awareness, acceptance, and homoeostasis expressed within the total being from the energy level to the material levels of behavior and cellular functions. The mechanisms of healing occur naturally. We can observe this in the body's intelligence in healing itself from an injury or in cases of spontaneous healing of an illness ordinarily considered terminal. (p. 52)

### Sound Therapy

Energetic healing is only one form used by healers. Look, for example, at the work of a nurse neuromuscular therapist and sound therapist Lynne Austin (2002):

> When a client comes to me and I am working on a specific tight muscle, sometimes the muscle will not relax under my hands. This is when I suddenly hear a tone or sound. I will repeat this tone as I am holding this body part, and I can feel my hand vibrate with the tone. I then know this is the appropriate sound, and whatever the intent is—for a muscle to relax, for the stiffness to leave, for a headache to go away—it will happen. The person is generally in awe that it worked and many times he feels the vibration as I do the tone. (p. 30)

Notice that both energy movement and use of sound involve some sense of a natural vibration accessible to the healer. The acupuncturist would also claim to be dealing with this natural energy in the form of *chi*.

Even healers who work primarily with the body assert that body and mind are inseparable. For example, nurse and rolfer (deep muscle massage) Bernau-Eigen (2002) says:

Where the body-mind comes together for me to work with, is at the
level of energy expression. I ask myself, where is expression moving
or held in the body? Then the question for me becomes where do I
focus my level of intervention: physical body, mind, emotion, or spirit?
I use the connection that works to access the healer within. (p. 79)

### Religious Healing

Not all healers come from the new paradigm. Healing has been associated with
religion for as long as history has been recorded. Laying-on of hands is the
term usually given to describe the method most often attributed to religious
miracle cures. Does the same process underlie both religious laying on of hands
and new paradigm energetic healing? There are those who believe so and others who prefer to think of religious healing as divine intervention. Here we'll
discuss another form of religious healing: prayer.

#### *Prayer*

Prayer is probably the most frequently used method in asking for help in a religious context. Gustafson (1998) defines prayer as

an intimate conversation of dialog between an individual and God or
a higher being. It is a practice common to all faiths and practiced by
persons in practically all societies. In addition to its importance as an
element in all organized religions, prayer is one of the oldest forms
of healing therapies. (p. 259)

Prayer is used by both the person with the problem and the professional
trying to help him. As MacNutt (1977), then Father MacNutt, said from the
perspective of the healer:

These saving actions of God include spiritual healings (such as being
freed instantly from long-standing alcoholism), emotional healings
(such as from schizophrenia and deep mental depression), and physical healings (such as growths disappearing in a matter of minutes).
For some these healings are immediate; for some they are gradual and
take months, and for still others nothing at all seems to happen. But
I would estimate that about 75 percent of the people we pray for, for
physical or emotional ailments, are either healed completely or experience a noticeable improvement. (p. 22)

Whether the impetus to heal is seen as arising from within the client or supplied from without by the healer, most healers agree that not everyone can be healed simply by an external intention. Many refer back to the purpose that the illness serves in a person's life, whether that refers to illness as teacher of an important lesson or even illness as secondary gain. MacNutt (1977) refers failures back to the will of God.

There is also the mystery of God's will . . . healing does not depend primarily upon prayer or spiritual power. Some people will not be healed because it is not God's will for them. (p. 98)

In the Buddhist tradition, Lama Surya Das (1999) says about healing:

In Buddhism, healing prayers take on special significance, because when we pray for healing, we pray for healing in the very largest sense. We ask not only that the being for whom we are praying will be cured of a specific disease or frame of mind. We are also praying that this being will be cured in the deepest ways that karma itself be expiated, purified, and exhausted. A Buddhist prayer for healing implies a petition that the entire life (or lifetimes) be healed, not just the temporary affliction. The deepest healing brings a return to spiritual as well as physical well-being. (p. 268)

All religions have some form of petitionary prayer, and all support the idea that petitionary prayer has the potential to be effective in healing. Other religious healing methods will be discussed in chapter 12.

## IMAGINATION AND INTENTION

Whether new paradigm or religious, healing seems to involve the factors of imagination and intention. In this case, imagination has nothing to do with "make believe," but, instead, with imaging, visualizing a desired outcome. Most healers believe that thought is the first step in bringing about a change in material reality (Barnum, 2002).

Intention is the second step after imaging a desired goal. In order to evoke intention, an intense attention to the task is required. Brooke Medicine Eagle (1989) gives a wonderful example of creating intention during a dance in a healing circle.

In doing this we have focused what we call a *first attention*—the everyday, physical body reality. With it we determine right from left, feel physical weight on one side of the body or the other, step down in rhythm with the drumbeat. . . .

Now I give a second-attention task: The dancers are to focus their attention on softening and opening the sole of the left foot, so that they have a growing sense of connection with Mother Earth below. (p. 59)

In the third attention, Brooke says one focuses not just on dancing and on Mother Earth, but extends outward until we include.

all the universes beyond us, encompassing those who have come before us and those who will come seven generations after us, until finally we embrace All Our Relations, All-That-Is. Such is an act of holiness.

This holiness is the essence of healing, which means to manifest wholeness in spirit and bring it into our bodies, our families, our communities, our world. We heal by beginning to consciously embody the Spirit that lives as one with us in all things. (p. 60)

Willing a goal into reality with imagination and intention, as one healer quotes (source unknown) can be summarized as: visualization plus vocalization equals manifestation. As one can easily perceive, imagination and intention appear to play significant parts in many forms of healing, both new paradigm and religious.

### TURF ISSUES

More and more one finds new paradigm healing in the nursing literature. Again the question is one of boundary: How is the new paradigm nurse healer different from other non-nurse healers? Nurses have always comprised a great portion of the healing community, but they haven't captured the turf, nor could they. How is nursing spiritualism different from the function of other healing spiritual leaders?

Whatever the results, we are left with the fact that the nurse and the healer use the same tactics. The similarity of the nurse's methods to that of other healers raises the boundary question as to the functions of nursing and of the healing community. The issue is whether nurses have left nursing when they heal (as opposed to cure) or whether what they are doing is nursing. Ironically, this is the same question that was once raised when nurse practitioners moved into primary care and were accused of practicing medicine.

Turf issues aside, the most important question for the purposes of this book is whether a conception of healing necessarily implies a spiritual interpretation, and the answer is no. Krieger (1981), for example, said:

Therapeutic Touch derives from, but is not the same as, the ancient art of the laying-on of hands. The major points of difference between Therapeutic Touch and the laying-on of hands are methodological; Therapeutic Touch has no religious base as does the laying-on of hands; it is a conscious, intentional act; it is based on research findings; and Therapeutic Touch does not require a declaration of faith from the healee (patient) for it to be effective. (p. 138)

The study of the movement of energies, as one illustration, is derived from what is called the subtle arts (because so many people are insensitive to their existence). Most schools teaching the subtle arts arise in religion or transpersonal psychology, both with inherent spiritual bases. However, one could just as easily take Krieger's position and assume that the movement of energies is simply a new science in the making.

## SUMMARY

The rapid growth of interest in healing is one of the more interesting facets of the new paradigm world-view. While nurses have been heavily involved in healing and healing therapies, the territory of healing is not owned by the nursing profession, nor is it likely to be. In the first place, many of the most successful healers aren't nurses, and the therapies associated with healing are not often taught in, or limited to, nursing programs.

Of course, many nurses who move into healing work come from programs where curricula stress holistic interpretations of the human being. While not all holistic theories embrace healing, most do, and most are grounded in the new paradigm.

In addition to new paradigm healers, there also are healers steeped in religious traditions. Virtually every religion has a healing tradition.

## REFERENCES

Austin, L. (2002). Interview. In B. S. Barnum, *The new healers: Minds and hands in complementary medicine* (pp. 24–36). Long Branch, NJ: Vista.

Barnum, B. S. (2002). *The new healers: Minds and hands in complementary medicine.* Long Branch, NJ: Vista.

Bernau-Eigen, M. (2002). Interview. In B. S. Barnum, *The new healers: Minds and hands in complementary medicine* (pp. 72–87). Long Branch, NJ: Vista.

Brennan, B. A. (1993). *Light emerging: The journey of personal healing*. New York: Bantam Books.

Brooke Medicine Eagle (1989). The circle of healing. In R. Carlson & B. Shield (Eds.), *Healers on healing* (pp. 58–62). New York: Jeremy P. Tarcher/Putnam Books.

Dossey, B. M. (1995). Dynamics of healing and the transpersonal self. In B. M. Dossey, L. Keegan, & C. E. Guzzetta (Eds.), *Holistic nursing: A handbook for practice* (2nd ed., pp. 39–57). Gaithersburg, MD: Aspen.

Dossey, B. M., Keegan, L., Guzzetta, C. E., & Kolkmeier, L. G. (Eds.). (1995). *Holistic nursing: A handbook for practice* (2nd ed.). Gaithersburg, MD: Aspen.

Gustafson, M. (1998). Prayer. In M. Snyder & R. Lindquist (Eds.), *Complementary/ alternative therapies in nursing* (3rd ed., pp. 259–268). New York: Springer.

Krieger, D. (1981). *Foundations for holistic health nursing practices: The renaissance nurse*. Philadelphia: J. B. Lippincott.

Lama Surya Das (1999). *Awakening to the sacred*. New York: Broadway Books of Random House.

Laurie, S. G., & Tucker, M. J. (1993). *Centering: A guide to inner growth*. Rochester, VT: Destiny Books.

MacNutt, F. (1977). *The power to heal*. Notre Dame, IN: Ave Maria Press.

McGlone, M. E. (1990, July). Healing the spirit. *Holistic Nursing Practice, 4*, 77–84.

Quinn, J. F. (1989, December). On healing, wholeness, and the Haelan Effect. *Nursing & Health Care, 10*, 552–556.

Quinn, J. F. (1994). Caring for the caregiver. In J. Watson (Ed.), *Applying the art & science of human caring* (pp. 63–71). New York: National League for Nursing Press.

Quinn, J. F. (2000). Transpersonal human caring and healing. In B. M. Dossey, L. Keegan, L. G. Kolkmeier, & C. E. Guzzetta (Eds.), *Holistic health promotion: A guide for practice* (3rd ed., pp. 37–48). Gaithersburg, MD: Aspen.

Schwartz, J. (2002). Interview. In B. S. Barnum, *The new healers: Minds and hands in complementary medicine* (pp. 50–63). Long Branch, NJ: Vista.

# PART V

## Spiritual Interventions in Health Care

**P**art V deals with the relationship of spiritual nursing therapies and the new paradigm and religion. In chapter 11, new paradigm approaches to therapy will be examined, and in chapter 12, a traditional religious approach to therapy will be discussed. A basic Judeo-Christian viewpoint will be taken here, recognizing that other religions have their unique styles of spiritual therapeutics. Brief references to Buddhism are included in both chapters, primarily because of the relationship to meditation. The reader wishing for a more comprehensive review of effects of culture and religions might review Spector's (1996) *Cultural Diversity in Health and Illness*. Techniques of spiritual care in the new paradigm and religion often are similar, but the explanations for their effectiveness are quite different.

Just what comprises a spiritual therapy? There are at least two perspectives one might take. First, one might examine therapies specifically designed to tend to that component of the human being identified as soul or spirit. Second, one could identify therapies arising from nursing theories in which spirituality plays a major part. In the second case, the therapy could be for something other than the spirit, most often the body. Most new paradigm theories blend aspects of body, mind, and spirit. What works for spirit also works for body and mind.

In every case, one must ask if the nurse qualifies for this work. Does she have the spiritual knowledge or the personal spiritual development required either to tend to the spirit or to tend to the whole person who is perceived with a spiritual component?

The nature of spiritual care calls into question not only the nurse's knowledge of spirit but her personal qualifications to offer spiritual guidance. Nagai-Jacobson and Burkhardt (1989) and Stuart, Deckro, and Mandle (1989) raised the problem of the nurse's potential spiritual deficiencies and the possible inadequacies of her spiritual resources. Their objections seem only fair. Few if any schools or employers take a measure of a nurse's spirituality, nor do many set about to equip her for providing spiritual care.

## REFERENCES

Nagai-Jacobson, M. G., & Burkhardt, M. A. (1989). Spirituality: Cornerstone of holistic nursing practice. *Holistic Nursing Practice, 3*(3),18–26.
Spector, R. E. (1996). *Cultural diversity in health & illness* (4th ed.). Stanford, CT: Appleton & Lange.
Stuart, E. M., Deckro, J. D., & Mandle, C. L. (1989). Spirituality in health and healing: A clinical program. *Holistic Nursing Practice, 3*(3), 35–46.

# Chapter 11

## Spiritual and New Age Therapeutics

### BODY-MIND-SPIRIT INTERFACE

As we saw in chapter 9, new paradigm theories often include an aspect of the human being that is primarily spiritual. Body-mind-spirit, transpersonal self, bio-psycho-social-spiritual being: however labeled, newer formulations of the human being have a spiritual component. Some theories, such as Newman's, make the very essence of the person spiritual, that is, evolving consciousness. The elements that are spiritual vary from theory to theory dependent on definitions of the human being.

As was said in the Introduction to Part V, two types of nursing are included among those listed as spiritual therapeutics: (1) methods for providing spiritual comfort or spiritual development, and (2) methods arising from a "spiritual" source but applied for other purposes, for example, body healing.

The methods applied to reach spiritual comfort/wisdom and to treat human illness in the New Age paradigm contrast sharply with the methods used under the scientific paradigm. Hypnotism, altered states of consciousness, and energy movement already have been mentioned. Other new (or revitalized) methods cover everything from yoga practices (Chang, 1963), to centering (Laurie & Tucker, 1993), to meditation techniques (LeShan, 1975; Odajnyk, 1993), to movement of energies associated with chakras and auras (Brennan, 1987, 1993; Pierrakos, 1990).

New paradigm theories assume that care of the spirit is a natural part of nursing. Yet care of the soul is a new and unexplored commitment for nursing. As might be expected with any new aspect of care, there is a need to explore the domain (in this case, the spiritual) before integrating it into nursing practice.

Over a decade ago, Clark, Cross, Deane, and Lowry (1991) called attention to the problem of nursing's inexperience with providing a spiritual dimension of care:

> The process of defining spiritual care and spiritual needs has been elusive at best. It is not sufficiently developed to provide students and practitioners clear direction in strategies for using it in an intervention or for measuring spirituality as a part of quality care. (p. 68)

Since this initial challenge, there has been much work done making spirituality a subject matter of nurses' attention. As we said earlier, the North American Nursing Diagnosis Association (NANDA, 1999–2002) even has a nursing diagnosis of spiritual distress. Numerous tools have been created to assess the patient's spirituality (see Burkhardt & Jacobson, 2000). Almost all efforts to deal with the spiritual closely resemble approaches used in assessing body and mind factors. In other words, the approach to the spiritual has been intellectual, with attempts to subject spirituality to measurement.

Still, we might credit this approach as an attempt to integrate spirituality into the patient's care. Nor when one looks at spirituality as an intellectual subject matter, is it surprising that the focus has been on assessment rather than on what to do once the assessment is complete. Recall the same order of development when the nursing process, along with nursing diagnosis, began. Early focus was all on diagnosis, only later moving on to related therapeutics.

### Diagnostic Variables

In seeking appropriate spiritual diagnoses, there have been attempts to isolate applicable variables. Often the same variables appear in both new paradigm and religious theories. The exploration of the variable *hope* was an early example. Today one finds the attempt to add diagnostic categories still ongoing. For example, one sees increasing work on the characteristic *serenity*. Roberts and Whall (1996) describe serenity as an awakened state implying harmony of body, spirit, and mind. It is, in their terms, "an outcome of development of the higher self" (p. 360). This definition places serenity in the new paradigm.

As is often the case, these authors describe and explain the spiritual variable comprehensively, although the nursing prescriptions attached to these explanations are problematic. When they grope for how to develop serenity in a client, they prescribe inspiring, guiding, and nurturing patients to seek lofty human values and to live with enhanced awareness of the present. These methods are more goals than processes, and one is still left wondering just what the nurse *does*.

## PSYCHOLOGICALLY ORIENTED SPIRITUAL THERAPIES

Many spiritual theories assume that the approach to aiding soul or spirit is one of talk and interaction. In other words, these theories handle the spiritual addition in the realm of interpersonal relationships.

Early on, Clark, Cross, Deane, and Lowry (1991) attempted to develop spiritual therapy:

> Spiritual well-being, the integrating aspect of human wholeness is characterized by meaning and hope. Quality care must include a spirit-to-spirit encounter between caregiver and patient. That includes the patient's acknowledgment of trust in the caregiver. (p. 68)

Notice that this orientation pushes us toward an interpersonal approach. Clark and colleagues identified five major spiritual interventions as reported by patients:

1. Establishing a trusting relationship
2. Providing and facilitating a supportive environment
3. Responding sensitively to the patient's beliefs
4. Integrating spirituality into the quality assurance plan
5. Taking ownership of the nurse's key role in the health care system (pp. 74–75)

Many would argue that four of these categories slip into psychology and common sense, while the remaining category (integrating spirituality into the quality assurance plan) avoids the question of just what spirituality means.

How does a spiritual encounter differ from a psychological one? Groping for the meaning of spirituality isn't easy. Indeed, spirituality may remain a word without universal definition as long as some associate it with traditional religion, others with an advanced level of human development, and yet others seeing spirituality as a growth beyond insular human existence.

Recall that in this book we have taken the spiritual to mean a person's search for, or expression of, his connection to a greater and meaningful context. For some people, that connection will be seen as a connection with God; for others it may be finding their place in the universe, and that may involve in-depth searching for a greater sense of self. A few interpersonal strategies of spirituality are illustrated below.

### Repatterning

Newman proposed a New Age therapy called repatterning (discussed more fully in chapter 9). Newman (2000) described repatterning in the following way:

> From the moment we are conceived to the moment we die, in spite of changes that accompany aging, we manifest a pattern that identifies us as a particular person: the genetic pattern that contains information that directs our becoming, the voice pattern that is recognizable across distances and over time; the movement pattern that identifies a person known to us a long way off even though no other features can be seen. These patterns are among the many explicate manifestations of the underlying pattern. It is the pattern of our lives that identifies us, not the substance that goes into making up that pattern. (p. 71)

In helping the patient to repattern, the nurse first must recognize the extant pattern, and that takes time. Nursing is a mutual coming together, a rhythm of relating, as Newman calls it, a process for which there cannot be specific steps or common goals. Further, the need to repattern occurs when the patient is in a state of chaos. Repatterning is bringing about a new and improved pattern, but the answer to what the nurse does cannot be prescribed except to say that it emerges within the dyadic relationship with the patient:

> The action indicated will become apparent only as the pattern becomes apparent. The action emerges from the "truth" discovered as clients find the center of their truth and discover the new rules that apply to their situations. Then *they* will know what to *do*. (p. 109)

Although she does not use the term *repatterning*, Watson's (1999) method, like Newman's, is an interpersonal one. Her motives appear to be more focused on the immediacy than on some ultimate change in the person, but like Newman, she focuses on the nurse's "ability to assess and realize another's condition of being-in-the-world and to feel a union with another" (p. 64).

Watson's method involves the entire self of the nurse. Watson (1999) labels her method *the art of transpersonal caring*, and its objective is to change the situation:

> The professional nurse differs from the patient or a friend in that the nurse helps integrate the subjective experience and emotions with the objective, external view of the situation. (p. 65)

Like Clark and colleagues, Watson and Newman apply techniques that are interpersonal emergents. These approaches primarily are linked to talking with a thinking patient.

### Regression Hypnosis

Hypnotic regression, or past life therapy, is used frequently in the new paradigm. Nurse psychotherapists often employ the tactic, either using hypnotism themselves or referring clients to an appropriate hypnotist. As mentioned in chapter 3, regression hypnosis has been used to reveal other lives, existence between life, and life early in the creation of the universe. Here we'll confine remarks to past life regression because that form is used for therapy, namely revealing the reasons for traumas that can't be attributed to events in the present life.

Use of regression hypnosis clearly implies a new paradigm belief in reincarnation, another concept imported from Eastern philosophies. Although the concept of reincarnation is ancient and has long been believed by most people in the world, its adoption in the Western world was achieved mainly under the new paradigm.

The need for regression presents itself in a patient who has unexplained mental or physical problems, conditions that do not seem to derive from any events in the present life. Nor is regression hypnosis the only access to such memories, although it is the most common one. As regressionist Weiss, MD (1992), says:

Most of my patients experienced past life regressions through hypnosis. However, others remembered previous lives through meditation, or spontaneously while experiencing intense déjà vu feelings, or through vivid dreams, or in other ways.

Many were able to rid themselves of chronic lifelong symptoms, such as specific phobias, panic attacks, recurrent nightmares, physical pain and illness, and so on. (p. 23)

Frequently, just finding the cause of present symptoms in a past life appears to be enough to remove symptoms in this life. Unresolved patterns appear to repeat in various lives, at least if one believes in a theory of reincarnation. Whether one completely understands and accepts the theory of reincarnation seems less important than the fact that the therapy has proved effective in many cases. One now finds past life hypnotists associated with major health care institutions.

## BODY-MIND SPIRITUALITY

In new paradigm beliefs, frequently the body is an access point for spirit. Indeed there is less differentiation of parts than was the case under the scientific paradigm. The therapies listed here deal with both body and mind in equal measures, and both are linked to spirit.

### Psychoneuroimmunoendocrinology

The approach known as *psychoneuroimmunoendocrinology* (PNIE) arose out of advances over the historical concept of psychosomatic disease. The effect of the mind on the body (and the notion of placebos) fell into place in this older model. Originally the focus was on the impact of the mind on the body. Only later did the model become more reciprocal with body effects on mind also important. We saw many syndromes described (e.g., the ulcer personality, heart attack-vulnerable "type A's," or the arthritic personality). Some of these syndromes since have been discounted. Sometimes the term *psychosomatic* became a negative label. "Her disease is psychosomatic," meaning, "It's all in her head." Placebos often fell under the same interpretation. When a person responded to a placebo, for example, his pain was judged as not real. None of the early mind–body work, however, had much, if anything, to do with spirituality.

Today's understanding of body–mind interfaces is much more sophisticated, with the newer term *psychoneuroimmunoendocrinology*. This new coinage replaces *psychosomatic*, and recognizes that more body systems are involved than the earlier term implied. Of course, psychoneuroimmunoendocrinology is an insane term that seeks to outdo antidisestablishmentarianism as the longest English word, but at least it stands for a credible concept. Sometimes endocrinology is omitted in the term. For example, Bartol and Courts (2000) refer to the concept as psychoneuroimmunology. In any case, the concept is simpler than the name. As Anderson (1997) defined it:

> Psychoneuroimmunoendocrinology is a way of framing the unity of mental, neurological, hormonal and immune functions with its many potential applications. PNIE addresses the influence of the cognitive images of the mind (whatever its elusive definition) on the central nervous system. And consequent interactions with the endocrine and immune systems. (p. 40)

Why, then, is PNIE related to spirituality? The reason has to do with the way such interfacing human systems work. In PNIE not merely the emotions (as tended to be perceived under the older term, psychosomatic) but also and specifically the cognitive functions of brain (and the belief structures that help organize cognition), can affect manifestations of disease. Hence, we can appreciate that the patient's spirituality (or lack of it) may help cause or cure illness. Indeed, we have come to appreciate the great complexity in interface of all human systems. Many studies now demonstrate the health promoting effects of having a firm spiritual compass. In the New Age, it is not particularly useful to differentiate body, mind, and spirit because they are intricately bound.

### Guided Imagery

Like PNIE, guided imagery uses the brain–body connection to foster good health. Post-White (1998), Schaub & Dossey (2000), and many other new paradigm nurses use guided imagery to treat illness. Guided imagery is possibly the second most popular new paradigm technique after therapeutic touch. Many people have a simplistic notion of guided imagery in which, for example, a patient imagines (visualizes) his body attacking and destroying the cancer cells. This is not to say that such simple imagery is not of value, but the technique has a more complex basis and more facets than the example illustrates. Post-White (1998) describes it this way:

> Although the scientific basis for how imagery and other mind–body interventions influence physiologic responses is in its infancy, there is evidence that there are biochemical connections between the brain and body and that mind-body interventions, such as imagery, can alleviate or control specific disorders. (p. 104)

This explanation closely relates guided imagery to PNIE.

Dossey (Dossey, Keegan, Guzzetta, & Kolkmeier, 1995) identifies numerous types of imagery including receptive, active, corrective biologic, symbolic, end-state, general healing, packaged, and customized imagery. These various types of imagery deal with various and diverse senses. Schaub and Dossey (2000) give an excellent review of the philosophy and research underlying guided imagery.

Although guided imagery is a specific use of imagery for healing, many in the new paradigm see imagery in a larger context, that of creating all of reality. As Zinn (2002) says:

> [e]verything imagined can become real. We manifest our reality, consciously and unconsciously, because of our imagination.

Elemental thought forms are the first step in creating reality. These thought forms stay alive by virtue of the energy put into them. A simple formula to follow is: the energic system plus consciousness equals the manifestation of form. (p. 66)

King, a non-nurse writer (1981), noted earlier that the potency of imagery —imagineering as he called it—arises because imagination precedes action:

Almost everything you have ever learned or experienced was preceded by imagination in some form or another. Even as a baby, though you may not remember it, you learned to crawl, walk, and run by first imagining yourself doing it and then following through. (p. 15)

Like so many other writers who deal with new paradigm phenomena, King placed imagery in a spiritual context, speaking of the part of the mind that imagines:

This part of your mind is also called the Higher Self, the god-self, Spirit, the Guardian Angel, and other terms intended to convey its basic nature. It isn't God, in the sense of the Ultimate Being, but it is the part of you that most directly knows God or the Universal Mind, and which acts as your channel for the power of life. (p. 51)

Although the active use of visual imagery is easy to understand, the unplanned arising of imagery during body work may be more complex. The notion that different parts of the body "hold" thoughts and memories is foreign to our Western notion that all emotions occur in the brain. Yet many new paradigm systems, for example, the Alexander technique and rolfing, claim that other tissues can hold memories and feelings. Take, for example, a case where a therapist used imagery to diagnose and treat a woman's severe depression following a burglary. As the patient talked about the event, the therapist systematically felt the major muscle groups of her body. The therapist felt the woman's neck and shoulders tense up when the woman complained that her husband had not taken proper precautions to safeguard their belongings.

The therapist asked the patient to become aware of how her neck and shoulder muscles felt at that moment, then asked the woman to think back to when she felt like that in the past. The woman took a few seconds, then began to cry as she recounted a time when she was very young and her father had let her down, failed to protect her from harm. The therapist then had both the physical and mental information necessary to work with the woman, releasing the memory through talk and massage. The cure involved both the muscle work and the talk work because the "memory," the image, was held in the neck and shoulders as well as in the mind.

Similarly, Bernau-Eigen (2002) speaks of imagery that arises for the client when she does physical body work:

> In all these systems of body work (Rolfing, Cranio-Sacral Therapy, and Visceral Manipulation), you access the interface of the body–mind complex. It is in conscious thinking that we speak of a body separate from a mind. However, I think that body and mind are one in the unconscious. Images similar to those which arise in dreams often arise for the client. They are gifts from the unconscious with which one can consciously communicate. (p. 78)

This example of spontaneous, emergent imagery is closer to the psychiatric technique of active imagination than to guided imagery in that imagery is planned in advance, with the outcome predetermined. Indeed, a popular form of guided imagery is termed *making affirmations* (e.g., "I am self-confident, I am attractive"). Like guided imagery, the goal is selected in advance, and the state is imagined.

Active imagination, in contrast, is not planned. Johnson (1986), who objects to the manipulations of guided imagery, said:

> The problem with these approaches to imagery is that it is the ego that does all the deciding. The unconscious is seen as a sort of stupid animal that has no viewpoint of its own, no wisdom to contribute. The whole point of the exchange is to train the unconscious to do what the ego wants. The ego's decisions may seem to be good ones; the problem is that the unconscious is not consulted in making them. (p. 186)

Johnson's notion, of course, deals primarily with psychoanalytic techniques, not with the patient trying to manipulate the end goal in relation to his cancer.

## Being and Doing

Because the approach of Dossey and colleagues involves both body and mind, it is placed under the body–mind label. Although their approach involves both being and doing, these elements are separate, not fused. In other words, the being activities do not evolve out of the doing activities or vice versa. They are used simultaneously.

As indicated in chapter 9, Dossey and Guzzetta's (2000) *doing* therapies include the more traditional nursing tasks, whereas *being* tasks use states of consciousness, including imagery, prayer, meditation, quiet contemplation, presencing, and intentionality (p. 11–15).

These authors also differentiated the sources of these two different methods as rational or paradoxical, with doing therapies falling into the rational linear healing, and being therapies falling into the paradoxical healing category, that is, happening without a scientific explanation. (pp. 16–17) Additional paradoxical therapies include biofeedback, placebos, miracle cures, and faith. Again, these therapies aim at body, mind, and spirit.

### Meditation

Although it involves the mind, meditation is included in body–mind spirituality because its attempt is not psychological, that is, it does not employ the intellect. Indeed, it tries to achieve the exact opposite: to turn off the continuously thinking brain. Meditation extends well beyond the psychological/spiritual relationship. Probably the most adopted method from Eastern cultures, meditation arises from a Buddhist tradition. Often it is employed for purposes other than spirituality, namely, stress reduction, lowering of blood pressure, promoting relaxation, or creating a general sense of well-being. Hence, meditation can be used either for health or spiritual concerns.

Laurie and Tucker (1993) describe meditation this way:

> [t]rue meditation, requires an emptying of the self. One closes the eyes, goes down to alpha level, and seeks the silence rather than something within or outside the self—in short, exhausting the mind as thoroughly as possible so that ideas, sounds, and sights are eliminated. . . . The stilling of the mind is the goal. (p. 86)

The attempt is to shut off the left-brain internal dialogue, to allow the right brain to come into dominance. Odajnyk (1993) differentiates two method of meditation, fixed and discursive:

> Fixed meditation aims at focusing the attention on a specific object, either internal or external. . . . Discursive meditation focuses the attention on a sequence of events: for example, reliving in one's imagination or through pictures the Passion of Christ; practicing some form of guided fantasy or Jung's technique of active imagination. (p. 48)

Maupin (1972) describes the technique and philosophy of meditation this way:

> Meditation is first of all a deep passivity, combined with awareness. It is not necessary to have a mystical rationale to practice meditation, but there are marked similarities in the psychological assumptions which underlie most approaches. The ego, or conscious self, is usually felt to be only a portion of the real self. The conscious striving, busy attempts to maintain and defend myself are based on a partial and misleading concept of my vulnerability, my needs, and the deeper nature of reality. In meditation I suspend this busy activity and assume a passive attitude. . . . Instead of diffusing myself in a welter of thoughts and actions, I can turn back on myself and direct my attention upstream to the outpouring, spontaneous, unpredictable flow of my experience. . . . (p. 220)

These brief reviews demonstrate the attempts to circumvent left-brain control, shifting the mind away from normal thought processes toward right-brain control. The right brain, of course, is the center for religious and spiritual experiences. Meditation is a learned skill, and the degree to which it alters one's state of consciousness varies with the skill of the practitioner.

Sometimes used by nurses (primarily those practicing psychotherapy), other Buddhist techniques include mindfulness and living in the present. These may be seen as part of meditation in some viewpoints. As Kabat-Zinn (1994) says:

> Mindfulness means paying attention in a particular way: on purpose, in the present moment, and nonjudgmentally. This kind of attention nurtures greater awareness, clarity, and acceptance of present-moment reality. (p. 4)

Methods aimed at spiritual relief have similar objectives, whether they emerge from traditional religion or the new paradigm. They aim to alleviate the stress that accompanies an illness, enhance the patient's coping ability, cure or mitigate an illness, decrease the patient's fear in facing death, or achieve in the patient a state of transcendence in which the outcome of the disease process is less important and, indeed, is surmounted by a spiritual recovery/enhancement.

### Bioenergetics

Movement of energy was discussed in chapter 10 as one mechanism of healing. Here we'll address energy movement as a technique used predominantly
for treating the body. Yet it is not always possible to separate soul work and
body work. As Hall (1997), a Reiki master, says:

> Reiki works on many levels of living things. The physical, mental,
> emotional and spiritual aspects are all enhanced with Reiki energy.
> (p. 7)

Many of the new paradigm therapies involve methods of moving energy
and altering the patient's energy field. The human energy field is conceived
as arising within and extending beyond the physical body in vibratory layers
of energy, visible to some persons but not to all, and termed *the human aura.*
These layers of being extend beyond the body that is researched in the scientific model. Those who claim the existence of these energy layers see them as
mediating numerous aspects of the person's existence (including health and
illness) that manifest in the aura before showing up in the physical body.

Major issues arise in energy work. First, of course, is the fact that the
whole notion requires a nontraditional conception of what comprises the human
being and whether the developing research has established the existence of
these energy fields. Where the existence of energy fields is accepted, the issue
becomes whether or not bioenergetics therapy is a spiritual system or simply
a new piece of scientific knowledge.

In fact, most people who work with bioenergetics see the system as a component of a spiritual world-view. However, the notion of bioenergetics could
be separated from this world-view, and some energy workers do that. Pierrakos
(1987) ponders this very question:

> Over my first twenty years of psychiatric work, developing through
> the bioenergetics approach, I found myself more and more concerned
> with the nature and innate functioning of the life force itself. I won-
> dered: What is this energy? Is it both substance and attribute, as yogic
> theory and the early Greeks saw it? Is it universal spirit, individual-
> ized somehow in matter, as viewed by the sixteenth-century physi-
> cian Paracelsus and the nineteenth-century poet Walt Whitman? Is it
> essentially material, either a self-contained electrodynamic system,
> as Yale biologist Harold Burr and his colleagues defined in it the
> 1930s, or else a variation of what Reich called the common func-
> tioning principle? Is it essentially spiritual, as religious thinkers and

healers from Buddha through Jesus to Pierre Teilhard de Chardin have conceived it? (p. 13)

When one grants the existence of an energy field around the human being, the next question to arise is whether that field can actually be manipulated by another person. Brennan (1987, 1993) asserts that we manipulate each other's energy fields in the course of our daily lives, whether or not we realize it.

For Brennan, a non-nurse healer, there are many levels to the human aura, and the ability to manipulate energy at those various levels depends on the practitioner's own evolution. The healer's own psychic and spiritual development allows her to refine her High Sense Perception. In other words, she develops the ability to discern different levels of the patient's being, each level finer (at a higher vibration level) than the level beneath it. Only when these levels are perceived through one or more of the senses can the healer work with them in full clarity and understanding. For Brennan, energy movement is a skill that develops as the healer develops.

On the other hand, Reiki practitioners (who have a somewhat different method of energy movement), say that the key lies in the practitioner's upper chakras being open rather than in some sort of High Sense Perception. Whatever the criteria, in almost every case, the psychic, spiritual, or brain wave state of the practitioner enters into the ability to move energy.

While most energy workers would grant that some untrained people have an instinctive and strong ability to move energy, most would not grant that the mechanical moving of one's hands over a patient's body—without the appropriate mental (state of consciousness) preparation, without knowledgeable control of energies through them—could be effective except in a serendipitous or accidental fashion.

The issues here are many, including: (1) whether the attempt to manipulate energy can be systematically effective apart from extensive training with verification of what the practitioner is doing, (2) whether or not the healer must herself have attained certain levels of personal development and/or requisite altered states of consciousness in which to exercise the skill, and (3) whether the attempt is always to give added energy or whether the attempt may be to give, remove, or balance energy as dictated by a client's condition.

### Therapeutic Touch

The most popular New Age energy manipulation in nursing is therapeutic touch, introduced to the field by Krieger (1981, 1993). One critical issue in this format is: Does therapeutic touch require the sort of High Sense Perception described by Brennan, or the assurance that their chakras are open as advocated by Reiki practitioners? Are any methods of validating the nurse's required mental status used? At present, therapeutic touch is sometimes taught to nurses as if it were a simple technique any willing nurse could learn in the space of a few hours, a technique not unlike taking a temperature.

Some would say that this perception short-circuits the actual process of energy movement. However they describe their procedures, most people who work with energy describe four major steps: (1) centering within oneself, so that one is detached from outside interference, thoughts, or negativities, (2) grounding oneself in an energy source outside of oneself in such a way that one can tap a universal energy, (3) focusing that energy through oneself into the patient, so as not to draw on one's own bodily energy, and (4) intention, that is, employing the will and affect so as to intend a good result for the patient.

Each of these steps requires significant skills if one believes the experts. The issue in nursing, then, is whether ineffectively trained nurses may in fact be creating no more than a placebo effect. All of this, of course, is not to deny the effective movement of energy, nor is it to say that all therapeutic touch is taught on a superficial level. Quinn (1994), for example, is clearly aware of the altered states required:

> At the start of a Therapeutic Touch session the nurse centers, that is, turns his or her attention inward, reaching a calm, relaxed, and open state of consciousness. In this state of consciousness, the Therapeutic Touch practitioner then consciously formulates the intent to be an instrument for helping or healing and focuses on wholeness and balance in the recipient. This process on the part of the Therapeutic Touch practitioner may be thought of as a repatterning of his or her own energy field in the direction of expanded consciousness, a consciousness experienced as unified, harmonious, peaceful, and ordered. (p. 66)

Shames and Keegan (2000) describe the phases of therapeutic touch as follows:

1. centering oneself physically and psychologically; that is finding within oneself an inner reference of stability
2. exercising the natural sensitivity of the hand to assess the energy field of the client for clues to differentiate the quality of energy flow
3. mobilizing areas in the client's energy field that appear to be nonflowing (i.e., sluggish, congested, or static)
4. directing one's own excess body energies to assist the client to repattern his or her own energies (p. 620)

Notice the difference from the prior formulation; here the transmitted energies are seen as being the nurse's "excess" body energies rather than tapping into a universal energy. Shames and Keegan credit this process to Krieger (1981), and they appear to agree about the transfer of energies. Krieger (1981) says about *prana* (energy):

> I saw the healer to be an individual whose personal health gave him or her access to an overabundance of *prana* (the healer's health being an indication that he or she was in highly efficient interaction with the significant field forces) and whose motivation and intentionality gave him or her a certain control over the projection of *prana* for the well-being of other. (p. 143)

In her later book, Krieger (1993) is less specific about the source of the energy transmitted. In speaking of her therapeutic touch model, she says:

> It does not delineate the treatment for the healee nor how healing might occur. Such issues demand a more heuristic approach than is now available with our present Western thinking, and of necessity they will have to be put aside at this time. However, you can take comfort in the thought that just as you do not need to know how a car works in order to drive it, so can you use Therapeutic Touch without knowing exactly how its healing processes operate. . . . (p. 111)

Whatever form of bioenergetics is used, the basics appear similar, albeit with slightly different techniques. Unlike therapeutic touch, in Brennan's process and Reiki, the energy exchange is proposed to draw upon a universal energy for which the healer becomes a channel. All healers agree, however, that they must center and ground themselves. This process may allow them to reach an altered state of consciousness, and, as we said earlier, pull energies from elsewhere *through* themselves rather than drawing on their own energies. Obviously, the healer's interpretation of what happens may differ from what is actually happening.

Alternately, one can propose that energy can be drawn either from a universal source or from one's own energy resources. Use of the latter may explain why some practitioners are fatigued by the process.

Another difference in viewpoints concerns a practitioner's need for sensitivity. As we said earlier, the healer's perception is critical in Brennan's model. Krieger (1993) also sees the practitioner as perceiving the energy need in the client:

In Therapeutic Touch, it is to the incessant flow of the healee's energy fields that you as the practitioner look when you are assessing the reality of the healee's condition. This reality is interpreted through indicators such as temperature differentials, pressure gradients, pulsations, "tingles," feelings similar to slight electric shocks, and so on. These indicators occur during the assessment and reassessment phases of Therapeutic Touch. (p. 108)

Shames and Keegan's second and third step in therapeutic touch involve a form of High Sense Perception, that is, the ability to sense the patient's state. Other healers speak of "intelligent energy" that will automatically distribute where it is needed without the practitioner having sensitive perception of the client's energy. Reiki practitioners, for example, grant that the energy will act correctly without direction or sensation on the part of the practitioner. Hall (1997) says:

With Reiki, you do not have to see the energy, nor concentrate on it at all. Nor do you remove energy from someone, or give them your energy. Reiki energy balances and harmonizes. If there is too much energy in an area, or if there is not enough, the area is out of balance: when there is imbalance, there is potential for illness. (p. 6)

All of these techniques of energy movement come under attack from the scientific paradigm, partly because they deal with body systems that are not found physically in today's research. Additionally, advocates may exaggerate claims of benefits derived, thereby hurting their own case. See, for example, Mathuna's (2000) criticism of therapeutic touch.

Other major new paradigm therapies, in addition to the ones discussed here, include relaxation therapy, music therapy, aroma therapy, laughter, thought field therapy, rolfing, reflexology, sound therapy, meditation, acupuncture, massage, or acupressure, among others.

The purpose of this book is not to teach New Age spiritual therapies but to note that these holistic therapies often are presented in a spiritual context, either as arising out of spiritual insights and information or as awakening or involving spiritual aspects of the patient in healing. Many of these therapies aim not merely at healing or treating a particular disease or injury, but also at creating greater self-awareness from a spiritual perspective.

## WHO IS THE THERAPIST: THE PRACTITIONER OR THE PATIENT?

With New Age therapies, another question arises: Who performs the therapies? The therapist, the patient, or both? Some techniques, such as acupressure and therapeutic touch, are procedures seen as being done *to* the patient. Other techniques, such as guided imagery, relaxation, meditation, and aroma therapy are seen as patient controlled. Even these patient-controlled therapies require teaching, however. Most commonly, the patient is seen as the final self-therapist, with the practitioner simply helping him access the therapeutic systems.

Another type of therapist is the medical mystic. We have already spoken about energy perceptions arising for some practitioners of energy movement. This, of course, is one type of medical assessment. In the case of medical mystics, the visions are even more definitive. As Myss (1996) describes her perceptions:

I gradually recognized that my perceptual abilities had expanded considerably. For instance, a friend would mention that someone he knew was not feeling well, and an insight into the cause of the problem would pop into my head. I was uncannily accurate. . . . (p. 1)

Like most medical mystics, Myss relates illness to spirit:

My particular insights, however, have shown me that emotional *and* *spiritual* stresses or dis-eases are the root causes of *all* physical illnesses. Moreover, certain emotional and spiritual crises correspond quite specifically to problems in certain parts of the body. (p. 6)

Stratton (1996) makes similar observations concerning her early developing abilities:

I turned around to see a woman standing in back of me. I asked her if she had a headache. Startled, she admitted she did. How did I know? I had just gotten it. (p. 19)

Stratton also relates her gift to the spiritual. For example, she says:

It is in this alchemical healing process that the physical body becomes a resurrected body. The old patterns and imprints die and make way for new life force to rise again. The body "remembers" wholeness, health, and its connection with God. (p. 160)

Some medical mystics, like Stratton, are also healers, working with energy movement where they find a disorder. Others serve simply as diagnosticians, often working with more traditional health practitioners.

## NEW AGE, RELIGION, AND SCIENCE: A RECONCILIATION?

Each major age (and its world-view) is eventually replaced by a new world-view with a differing perception of reality. While negating the receding world-view, the new paradigm incorporates much of the old view into itself. Hence, in the present shift one finds New Age practitioners attempting to use rigorous scientific inquiry (the method of the scientific paradigm) to validate the effectiveness of their practices.

Certainly there is no sign that New Age practitioners (from nurses to healers) wish to negate the work of science, including modern medicine. Instead, the view is that the scientific model and scientific methods work extremely well for a certain mid-range of phenomena. But in the new paradigm there are phenomena lying outside of that range that do not lend themselves to interpretation or investigation by the accepted methods of the scientific model.

Scientists' tactics, when faced with such phenomena, have been to ignore them, casting each phenomenon as a human failing—imaginary, hysterical, or wish fulfilling. Scientists who choose to study such phenomena often find themselves stigmatized by their colleagues, under as much censure as earlier scientists who once wanted to investigate whether the earth could possibly be rotating around the sun.

There are certain New Age therapies, such as hypnosis and acupuncture, that have reached a high degree of acceptance within the scientific world, but the acceptance is often grudging. Other therapies, as we said earlier of therapeutic touch, are under attack for poor science. When such techniques are accepted by those working in the scientific paradigm, it is because of overwhelming evidence that they work, not because the explanatory paradigm has been accepted.

Much of this book has drawn a dividing line between New Age spirituality and spirituality arising in traditional religions. It is true that they pose radically different views of reality. Yet both of these views conflict with the scientific world-view. They often are written off in the scientific model with the same stroke of the pen or computer as mere wish fulfillment and fuzzy thinking.

Yet, as the rising paradigm indicates, man is no longer content to repress all of the spiritual and non-objective elements of his being and his sense of reality. The absence of a spiritual element ultimately makes the human being less. The issue is one of how far the pendulum will swing in reinventing of the world. Will the next era sustain a continuing contest between science and the new paradigm? Or will a positive synthesis of the best of science and the new paradigm emerge?

## SUMMARY

Spiritual therapeutics are beginning to reappear in nursing practice. Some of the therapies represent a renewal of earlier religious practices; others are new paradigm therapies, often involving manipulation of the nurse's or the patient's state of consciousness. Because the latter are still relatively new on the scene, their effectiveness requires continued study.

Many of these new paradigm practices are associated with a spiritual philosophy or system of belief. Typically the belief systems come closer to Eastern philosophies than to traditional Western ones.

At least two factors are at play in new paradigm effects on nursing therapy: (1) acceptance of spirituality as a valid source of nursing processes with patients, and (2) the need to learn new procedural ways and means for implementing spiritual therapies. Naturally, these changes bring with them all the adjustment required when any new way of behaving enters nursing.

## REFERENCES

Anderson, R. A. (1997, October). Psychoneuroimmunoendocrinology. *Townsend Letter for Doctors & Patients, 171*, 40–41.

Bartol, G. M., & Courts, N. G. (2000). The psychophysiology of bodymind healing. In B. M. Dossey, L. Keegan, & C. E. Guzzetta (Eds.), *Holistic nursing: A handbook for practice* (3rd ed., pp. 69–88). Gaithersburg, MD: Aspen.

Bernau-Eigen, M. (2000). Interview. In B. S. Barnum, *The new healers: Minds and hands in complementary medicine* (pp. 73–87). Long Branch, NJ: Vista.

Brennan, B. A. (1987). *Hands of light: A guide to healing through the human energy field*. New York: Bantam Books.

Brennan, B. A. (1993). *Light emerging: The journey of personal healing*. New York: Bantam Books.

Burkhardt, M. A., & Jacobson, M. G. N. (2000). Spirituality and health. In B. M. Dossey, L. Keegan, & C. E. Guzzetta (Eds.), *Holistic nursing: A handbook for practice* (3rd ed., pp. 91–121). Gaithersburg, MD: Aspen.

Chang, G. (1963). *Teachings of Tibetan yoga*. New Hyde Park, NY: University Books.

Clark, C., Cross, J. R., Deane, D. M., & Lowry, L. W. (1991). Spirituality: Integral to quality care. *Holistic Nursing Process, 5*(3), 67–76.

Dossey, B. M., & Guzzetta, C. E. (2000). Holistic nursing practice. In B. M. Dossey, L. Keegan, & C. E. Guzzetta (Eds.), *Holistic nursing: A handbook for practice* (3rd ed., pp. 5–26). Gaithersburg, MD: Aspen.

Dossey, B. M., Keegan, L., Guzzetta, C. E., & Kolkmeier, L. G. (Eds.). (1995). *Holistic nursing: A handbook for practice* (2nd ed.). Gaithersburg, MD: Aspen.

Hall, M. (1997). *Practical reiki: A practical step by step guide to this ancient healing art.* San Francisco: Thorsons, an imprint of Harper/Collins.

Johnson, R. A. (1986). *Inner work: Using dreams and active imagination for personal growth.* San Francisco: HarperSan Francisco.

Kabat-Zinn, J. (1994). *Wherever you go there you are: Mindfulness meditation in everyday life.* New York: Hyperion.

King, S. (1981). *Imagineering for health.* Wheaton, IL: Theosophical Publishing House.

Krieger, D. (1981). *Foundations for holistic health nursing practices: The renaissance nurse.* Philadelphia: J. B. Lippincott.

Krieger, D. (1993). *Accepting your power to heal: The personal practice of therapeutic touch.* Santa Fe, NM: Bear.

Laurie, S. G., & Tucker, M. J. (1993). *Centering: A guide to inner growth* (2nd ed.). Rochester, VT: Destiny Books.

LeShan, L. (1975). *How to meditate.* New York: Bantam Books.

Mathuna, D. P. (2000). Evidence-based practice and reviews of therapeutic touch. *Journal of Nursing Scholarship, 32*(3), 279–285.

Maupin, E. W. (1972). On meditation. In C. T. Tart (Ed.), *Altered states of consciousness* (3rd ed., pp. 217–240). San Francisco: HarperSanFrancisco.

Myss, C. (1996). *Anatomy of the spirit: The seven stages of power and healing.* New York: Three Rivers.

Newman, M. A. (2000). *Health as expanding consciousness* (2nd ed.). Boston: Jones and Bartlett.

North American Nursing Diagnosis Association (1999–2002). *Nursing diagnoses: Definitions and classification, 2001–2002 (4th ed.).* Philadelphia: NurseCom.

Odajnyk, V. W. (1993). *Gathering the light: A psychology of meditation.* Boston: Shambhala.

Pierrakos, J. C. (1990). *Core energetics: Developing the capacity to love and heal.* Mendocino, CA: LifeRhythm Publication.

Post-White, J. (1998). Imagery. In M. Snyder & R. Lindquist (Eds.), *Complementary/ alternative therapies in nursing* (3rd ed., pp. 103–122). New York: Springer.

Quinn, J. (1994). Caring for the caregiver. In J. Watson (Ed.). *Applying the art and science of human caring* (pp. 63–71). New York: National League for Nursing Press.

Roberts, K. T., & Whall, A. (1996, Winter). Serenity as a goal for nursing practices. *Image, 28*(4), 359–364.

Schaub, B. G., & Dossey, B. M. (2000). Imagery: Awakening the inner healer. In B. M. Dossey, L. Keegan, & C. E. Guzzetta (Eds.), *Holistic nursing: A handbook for practice* (3rd ed., pp. 539–581). Gaithersburg, MD: Aspen.

Shames, K. H., & Keegan, L. (2000). Touch: Connecting with the healing power. In B. M. Dossey, L. Keegan, & C. E. Guzzetta, (Eds.), *Holistic nursing: A handbook for practice* (3rd ed., pp. 613–635). Gaithersburg, MD: Aspen.

Strahon, E. K. (1996). *Touching spirit: A journey of healing and personal resurrection.* New York: Simon & Schuster.

Watson, J. (1999). *Nursing: Human science and human care: A theory of nursing.* Boston: Jones and Bartlett.

Weiss, B. L. (1992). *Many lives, many masters: Through time into healing.* New York: Simon & Schuster.

Zinn, L. (2002). Interview. In B. S. Barnum, *The new healers: Minds and hands in complementary medicine* (pp. 64–71). Long Branch, NJ: Vista.

# Chapter 12

## Spirituality, Traditional Religion, and Traditional Therapeutics

New Age therapeutics were not the first spiritual interventions on the scene. For generations, in the Judeo-Christian tradition, nurses used religious efforts in treating patients. Early on, caregivers may have felt that spirituality was the only component of the human being over which they had some control. Further, spirituality or soul was accepted as part of the human being with little question. As Armstrong (1993) said, even in our times:

> [h]uman beings are spiritual animals. Indeed, there is a case for argu-
> ing that *Homo sapiens* is also *Homo religiosus*. Men and women
> started to worship gods as soon as they became recognizably human;
> they created religions at the same time as they created works of art.
> This was not simply because they wanted to propitiate powerful forces;
> these early faiths expressed the wonder and mystery that seem always
> to have been an essential component of the human experience of this
> beautiful yet terrifying world. Like art, religion has been an attempt
> to find meaning and value in life, despite the suffering that flesh is
> heir to. (p. xix)

Among the traditional spiritual therapies were prayer, contemplation, fasting and other methods of self-temperance, music, chanting, encouraging the patient in his faith, arranging for religious rites, spiritual counseling, reading the Bible or other religious materials, praying for or with the patient, worshiping, and discussing and seeking the purpose and meaning of life.

Religion has long been a source of strength for people, especially those undergoing health crises. Indeed, religion is undergoing a resurgence as the inadequacy of mere psychological approaches becomes evident. We seek for something more in trying to understand ourselves. As Hillman (1996) said:

To uncover the innate image we must set aside the psychological frames that are usually used, and mostly used up. They do not reveal enough. They trim a life to fit the frame; developmental growth, step by step, from infancy, through troubled youth, to midlife crisis and aging, to death. Plodding your way through an already planned map, you are on an itinerary that tells you where you have been before you get there, or like an averaged statistic foretold by an actuary in an insurance company. The course of your life has been described in the future perfect tense. (p. 5)

This view reflects the paucity of values that many find in the limiting scientific paradigm. One recourse to this paucity is found, worldwide, in religion. Moore (1994) commented on this vacuity and religion's ability to fill it:

Another aspect of modern life is a loss of formal religious practice in many people's lives, which is not only a threat to spirituality as such, but also deprives the soul of valuable symbolic and reflective experience. Care of the soul might include a recovery of formal religion in a way that is both intellectually and emotionally satisfying. One obvious source of spiritual renewal is the religious tradition in which we were brought up. (p. 212)

Moore (1994) described the benefits of religious ritual, the comfort of the familiar pattern, the repetitive renewal and remembrance:

Spiritually doesn't arrive fully formed without effort. Religions around the world demonstrate that spiritual life required constant attention and a subtle, often beautiful technology by which spiritual principles and understanding are kept alive. For good reason we go to church, temple, or mosque regularly and at appointed times: it's easy for consciousness to become lodged in the material work and to forget the spiritual. Sacred technology is largely aimed at helping us remain conscious of spiritual ideas and values. (p. 204)

## TRADITIONAL NURSING THERAPIES FOR SPIRITUAL NEEDS

This section focuses on Judeo-Christian practices simply because these are the ones most likely to find an accord between nurse and patient in our society. When a patient has a different religious orientation, the nurse's task is more challenging. Often it involves gaining the assistance of appropriate religious

leaders from the patient's own orientation. Six basic religious nursing therapies will be discussed here: (1) prayer, (2) presencing, (3) religious contemplation, (4) ritual, (5) giving meaning to illness and suffering, and (6) helping
the patient maintain faith.

### Prayer

Prayer is the most frequent of the traditional nursing spiritual therapies. It is
a flexible measure because the nurse can pray for a patient without telling anyone, including the patient. Praying with a patient is a variant used when there
is agreement to do so by both parties.

Taylor and Ferszt (1990) gave a creative way to fit prayer into a busy work
schedule:

> [o]ne technique that we have found helpful is to repeat a phrase from
> the Psalms 46:10: "Be still and know that I am God." We take the
> phrase and delete the last word until we are left with the word "Be."
> (p. 37)

This exercise (dropping a word with each repetition) has an interesting
effect that the authors claim "take(s) only a minute but that is often enough
time to remind us to slow down and to remember that we are not alone in our
lives and our work" (p. 37). In this case, the prayer may be used for the nurse
herself as much as for the patient.

As was the case with various New Age therapies, there are now numerous studies on the efficacy of prayer, usually measured in terms of quicker
recovery, or in mortality and morbidity statistics. In both cases (New Age therapies and religious prayer) people committed to the scientific paradigm have
difficulty accepting positive study conclusions and often, sometimes with reason, criticize the study methodologies. As in this case, it is interesting to see
the scientist's own research tools being applied to "off bounds" religious and
new paradigm subject matters.

Medicine developed many advocates of "religiosity" and techniques such
as prayer as means to better healing. Matthews (1997) typified the conclusions
draw from research into the relationship of health and religion:

> [a]ddressing religious variables in medical settings may have posi-
> tive effects for patients as well as the health care profession. Since
> physicians and other health care professionals are charged with guard-
> ing and promoting public health, and since data from a variety of

sources are beginning to point to the value of religious commitment upon health, it may become important, necessary, and ethical for physicians, and appropriate for federal health policy, to begin to support, and even perhaps to encourage such commitment. (p. 5)

### Presencing

Presencing is the nurse's simply being with the patient in a meaningful human way. McKivergin (2000) described presencing as:

The essence of presence, "being with," implies a conscious intention to appreciate the connection of the moment. A moment in time, the reality of the shared experience in the "now," creates an open container through which life, energy, and healing can flow. (p. 210)

Donley (1991) warned that physical presencing is not enough without "enter(ing) into the reality of the suffering so that a sense of communion and solidarity with the sufferer develops" (p. 179). She observes that in nursing practice, presence may be perceived as passivity, and high technology can work against compassionate presence. Donley's (1991) work (in a Roman Catholic tradition) focused on the patient, specifically his suffering:

Nursing's response to suffering persons runs parallel to the religious tradition: accompaniment, meaning giving and action. Presence at the bedside, a traditional value, is expressed by words as bedside nurse or "hands on" nursing. There are literary, artistic, and historic accounts of nurses sitting with and quietly comforting suffering persons. (p. 181)

Taylor and Ferszt (1990) said of presencing:

We have found that when we view our work with the dying as "accompanying" them on their journey, and not running away from them physically or emotionally, facing death is easier. (p. 35)

One finds a similar concern is expressed at Calvary Hospital in the Bronx, New York, where the term *accompaniment* is often used interchangeably with presence, although one could argue that they are discrete variables. At Calvary, focus is also placed on yet another formulation of the concept, that is, *non-abandonment*. Cimino (1984), one of the physicians instrumental in instilling this particular value at Calvary, put it this way in addressing a group of graduating physicians:

Being ill is a frightening experience, and care in a hospital can be so impersonal it enhances this fear. "Non-abandonment" goes beyond the usual standards of legal negligence. It means removing this aura of fear. You must encourage communication, show genuine concern, be available, keep your promises, and when you change services, this next year, ensure the patients' continuity of care with the next physician. (p. 4)

One of the problems for nurses in accepting a strategy of presencing, accompaniment, or non-abandonment, is the fact that it may not involve "doing" something. Indeed, it may involve just the opposite: sitting quietly, holding a patient's hand. With the pressure that nurses feel when they are not "busy," simply accompanying patients may leave nurses feeling frustrated, sensing that they are not tending to assigned tasks. The lack of time for such valid patient needs as presencing is, unfortunately, a hallmark of today's practice. Baer, Fagin, and Gordon (1996) discuss the abandonment of the patient in terms that bring this deficit home.

### Religious Contemplation

Religious contemplation is much like New Age meditation. Both of these activities alter the state of consciousness. As used here, contemplation refers to the extensive use of time for considering/envisioning phenomena beyond one's personal life concerns. Although contemplation may involve different subject matters, religious contemplation still tops the list. Contemplation is also used in shamanic vision quests and in various guided meditations. Deikman (1972) described contemplation in the following way:

Contemplation is, ideally, a nonanalytic apprehension of an object or idea—nonanalytic because discursive thought is banished and the attempt is made to empty the mind of everything except the percept of the object in question. . . . The renunciation of worldly goals and pleasures, both physical and psychological, is an extension of the same principle of freeing oneself from distractions that interfere with the perception of higher realisms or more beautiful aspects of existence. (p. 39)

The term *contemplation* is sometimes taken as synonymous with meditation. More often, it is seen as a special type of discursive meditation that focuses on guided visualization. As Maupin (1972) stated:

Meditation has been used in the Western sects of Christianity. Roman Catholicism appears to have articulated a psychology, or map, of what happens with meditation. The conscious exercise of attention leads to a spontaneous flow of experience to which the person becomes a receptive onlooker. At its extreme, the feeling of a separate self is lost and union with the object of meditation is felt. This state is called contemplation. (p. 217)

Maupin pointed out the technique for applying contemplation to religion:

[t]he reader is led to imaging what Christ or Mary or various saints were experiencing at crucial points in their careers. (p. 217)

Johnson (1986) described the process this way:

In this guided imagery you go, for example, to the Via Dolorosa. It is the day of the Crucifixion, and you are there, present in your imagination. You smell the dust, sweat, and blood. You hear the jeering of the crowd. You see the crown of thorns, the cross, the blood flowing. You feel the sharp stones beneath your feet, the sun beating down on you as you move with the crowd toward Golgotha.

   In this way . . . the events of the life of Christ were made so vivid—smelling, feeling, touching, hurting—that they became actual, immediate experiences. This sort of guided imagery is good if it truly serves your religious purposes. It was geared mainly to the medieval mentality, but much of that mentality still lives on in us and we can honor it. (p. 187)

Maupin's and Johnson's descriptions of contemplation are not exclusive to Christianity but are used by other religions as well, each guiding the contemplative as to what he is to imagine.

George's (1995) description reinforces the interplay between contemplation and religion:

It should not be forgotten that the techniques of contemplation and renunciation are exercised within the structure of some sort of theological schema. This schema is used to interpret and organize the experiences that occur. (p. 41)

Most religions are bifurcated into two paths: (1) a primarily "left brain" experience—that experienced by most members, and (2) a mystic tradition followed by a small portion of members and clergy. The first path, although primarily left-brained, can be accompanied by positive emotions, including awe and appreciation, but all thoughts and feelings arise out of what is learned. The second path involves direct, personal experiences. Clergy have used contemplation to promote the occurrence of mystic encounters for centuries. Now the practice is becoming more popular among lay members as well.

Contemplation need not be associated with religious goals, but it usually is. For many generations, free time for contemplation was found primarily in a religious life. Even the term *contemplative* usually refers to a sequestered religious devotee. Furthermore, a religious life encourages contemplation directed beyond one's personal concerns. As Borchert (1994) said:

> The contemplative form of mysticism has always been rather elitist, fit only for monks who have been granted an opportunity for it. It was not considered suitable for people with lots of things to attend to. (p. 42)

Even the use of imagery (a new paradigm technique) has its equivalent in religion. Taylor and Ferszt (1990) adapted the technique of imagery to serve a religious purpose:

> We have often found that religious imagery has been therapeutic for us as well as for our patients. Imaging God, the Higher Power, or the reality of love surrounding not only the patient or family but also us as we care for others has been helpful, especially when we are not physically doing something for the patient or family but are "being with them." (p. 34)

## Ritual

Ritual is the repetition of a valued series of thoughts and/or actions. When a positive pattern recurs with regularity, it is entrained in the brain in a unique fashion, awakening familiarity, belonging, and associated emotive responses. Every religion uses rituals from its holy days, to celebrations, to routine services, to patterns of behavior expected from its members. (Some authors differentiate between rites and rituals, but we will not delve into these fine points.)

Patients may be uncomfortable when removed from access to comforting religious rituals, even when an illness makes such rituals impossible. When these circumstances occur, the subject should be discussed so that the patient does not feel stressed by this necessary but usually temporary change. The nurse may be able to arrange for some level of replication within the health care facility. Chaplaincy programs have application of familiar ritual as one of their aims.

Ritual is an important element in separating a generalized spirituality from religious spirituality. It is possible for a person to be spiritual without invoking ritual, but religions always apply rituals. Rituals may be individual or shared, but religious rituals are usually shared, building a sense of community and belonging. Most worship services take the form of ritual, with both the advantages and limitations that offers. The advantage is that the deity may be addressed in terms that have a "stamp of approval," as well as being comforting in their familiarity. The limitation, of course, is that the worship format may be completed in a mindless fashion, without attention to what is said.

Moore (1994) described ritual in the following way:

> Ritual maintains the world's holiness. Knowing that everything we do, no matter how simple, has a halo of imagination around it and can serve the soul enriches life and makes the things around us more precious, more worthy of our protection and care. (p. 228)

Spector (1996) marked the history of ritual and its function in early times, that is to protect vulnerable tribes and individuals from evil in various perceived forms. When a ritual was believed to be effective, it was institutionalized, repeated, and, later, often absorbed into developing religions, where its form might be changed to accommodate the religious beliefs. One sees religious ritual, for example, using a rosary, as a modern equivalent in which the ritual is employed to ward off threats to one's health or to improve one's chances of recovery.

Moore (1994) also notes that pathological ritual, for example, in obsessive-compulsive disorder, may signal a lack of soul-nourishing ritual for which we long.

### Giving Meaning to Illness and Suffering

When searching for meaning in suffering, Donley (1991) noted the many possible meanings that might be attached to suffering, including punishment, mystery, and redemption. Although different religious authorities might disagree on the meaning of suffering, most perceive it as a potential stimulus toward some greater good (however defined) if the patient has the strength to use the suffering in the "right" manner.

To what degree a nurse can help a patient find meaning in suffering depends on so many variables that it is very difficult to predict success or failure. What is the nurse's own spiritual state and the security of her religious beliefs? To what degree is the patient open to spiritual or religious suggestions? To what degree does he consider a nurse an appropriate person for a role like seeking meaning? To what degree does a patient seek meaning in his condition?

Disease and illness have often been the sources of suffering. In a religious context, one goal of growth may be salvation. Peck (1993) noted an interesting relationship between salvation and healing:

> [t]he word *salvation* means "healing." It comes from the same word as *salve*, which you put on your skin in order to heal an area of irritation or infection. Salvation is the process of healing and the process of becoming whole. And health, wholeness, and holiness are all derived from the same root. (p. 25)

In assessing suffering from a spiritual perception, Donley (1991) finds it important to differentiate between pain and suffering. She sees pain as a physical response to injury, while suffering fills a larger context:

> Suffering can be dehumanizing. Concern for the spiritual well-being of others requires attention to those forces and factors that can diminish the spirit. Suffering can be one of these forces. (p. 179)

This thought indicates that suffering can have divergent effects, from promoting spiritual growth to diminishing the human spirit. In relation to the suffering patient, then, it is important that the nurse assess the patient's response. Even when suffering is perceived as a valid path to spiritual or religious growth, relief of suffering is considered a worthy goal by almost everyone drawn to care for the sick. As Donley (1991) says, passive endurance is not a Christian response.

The concept of suffering is also critical in the Buddhist tradition. Indeed, suffering is sometimes seen as a condition of living rather than associated only with occasional illness, as is the usual orientation in this society. As Thich Nhat Hanh (1998) says:

> There are many practices that can help us face our suffering, including mindful walking, mindful breathing, mindful sitting, mindful eating, mindful looking, and mindful listening. One mindful step can take us deep into the realization of beauty and joy in us and around us. (p. 39)

Mindfulness, living in the present, and meditation were addressed under new paradigm practices, but they originated in, and are still a vital part of, Buddhist religious practice.

### Helping the Patient Maintain Faith

Faith is an important spiritual therapy for many patients. For others, faith may be questioned as they respond with anger, a sense of betrayal or loss, or a sense of indignant unfairness in relation to their illnesses. Indeed, loss of faith has been discussed as a nursing problem by many groups building nursing diagnosis systems.

Maintaining faith may have much to do with resolving the perceptions of betrayal, loss, or unfairness. At times, it may be appropriate for the nurse to explore these feelings with the patient. Yet, ultimately, faith (or its restoration) cannot be achieved by reasoning because faith is not a matter of knowledge. As Armstrong (1993) said:

> Faith did not mean assent to the propositions of a creed and it was not "belief" in orthodox opinion. Instead, faith was a leap in the dark toward a reality that had to be taken on trust. (p. 278)

Taylor and Watson (1989) quote the case of Job from the *Bible:*

> The suffering of Job epitomizes the individual's tenacity in the face of seeming irrational suffering. Job's friends attempt to convince him that the reason for his suffering lies in some offense he has committed and is thus a punishment wrought on him, but Job maintains his own righteousness and innocence and cries out against the inequities of Yahweh's wrath. . . . Two other answers emerge: The prolog suggests that Job's suffering is a test of his faith. The epilog suggests that suffering has a redemptive capacity. By accepting his suffering with continued faith, Job is brought into a restored state. (p. 14)

Maintenance of faith is the most controversial of nursing therapies. It assumes that religious faith is always a value to be maintained. A simplistic notion of maintaining faith, for example, might promote premature closure of the sort of seeking that moves a person from Peck's (1993) Stage Two level of religious development (formal/institutional religion, characterized by submission to the rules) to Stage Three (rebellion from unthinking submission, often resulting in doubters, atheists, and agnostics). Hence, a loss of faith might actually open a channel to more serious inquiry into the meaning of religion in one's life, albeit not a search that will necessarily be answered on the nurse's watch.

## MATTERS OF CONSCIENCE

It is impossible to talk about nursing therapies without mentioning the necessity for the nurse to be faithful to her own religious convictions and/or her conscience, however derived. Although we tend to think of conscience as something tied to a religion, that is far from required. Atheists and agnostics have their own developed senses of right and wrong, and no work situation should require any nurse to perform an act that goes against his or her individual conscience.

This can be a problem for an individual if the system pressures him or her to act in ways felt as wrong. It becomes an organizational problem: the nursing organization must see that procedures are created allowing nurses to withdraw from practices that go against their beliefs and consciences.

The key issues of conscience today are little changed from those of past eras: the notion of assisted suicide, the possibility of death as a side effect from narcotic pain control, and rights and wrongs of abortion. New technology continues to add to the unique problems of conscience as well. For example, issues of cloning and use of cells from aborted fetuses are prominent at present.

## RELIGIOUS COUNSELORS

Ensuring that the patient has access to the appropriate religious authorities is part of meeting the responsibility for religious therapy. Most large institutions have regular systems of access, often including in-house chaplaincy services. Whether or not chaplaincy programs are available, the nurse should inquire as to the patient's religious preferences and needs and alert appropriate religious sources.

The nurse must recognize the importance religious ceremony may hold in the patient's life. Unfortunately, the nursing literature tends to be glib and simplistic concerning religious needs (or what religion can provide) for the person faced with a set of stresses. Although last rites is the most frequently encountered requirement, others rites may assume equal significance. Just having a priest, rabbi, minister, or other religious leader visit may be very uplifting to many patients. Spector's book (1996) addresses many of these religious preferences.

## NEW AGE AND RELIGIOUS THERAPIES: THE SAME OR DIFFERENT?

Many parallels can be found between new paradigm and religious therapies. The laying-on of hands by a religious healer, for example, is not unlike therapeutic touch or other forms of bioenergetics. The technique is not so much different as is the motivation. In a religious context, laying-on of hands is seen as conveying the Lord's power and will through the healer. In the New Age paradigm, therapeutic touch is often related to a new paradigm conceptualization of spirituality, often one of a universal power or energy, Tao, or some formulation of God. It is also possible to see these energies as purely scientific—a domain open for further scientific inquiry. As Krieger (1981) said about therapeutic touch:

> Therapeutic Touch derives from, but is not the same as, the ancient art of the laying-on of hands. The major points of difference between Therapeutic Touch and the laying-on of hands are methodological; Therapeutic Touch has no religious base as does the laying-on of hands; it is a conscious, intentional act; it is based on research findings; and Therapeutic Touch does not require a declaration of faith from the healee (patient) for it to be effective. (p. 138)

There are other similarities between the new paradigm and religion. One finds, for examples, rituals created in the new paradigm just as one sees in religion. Summer solstice and full moon may replace Christmas, Easter, and Hanukkah as sources for celebration. Chanting ohm may replace crossing oneself, but the ritual element remains. Similarly, meditation and religious contemplation call on the same processes, and religious prayers are similar to new paradigm affirmations.

### RELIGION AND THE NURSE

In addition to the patient, one needs to consider the religious needs of the nurse. Nurses also face stresses. They need recourse to a perspective that will bring meaning and comfort in the situation. Concerning the nurse, Kerfoot (1995) said:

> [m]any who went into health care for altruistic reasons before health care became a business are feeling a sense of anxiety and are experiencing a deep chasm between the demand and necessity for profitability and the need for meaning and growth in one's life. (p. 49)

Traditional religions offer such meaning and solace. Taylor and Ferszt (1990) described the needs of nursing staff for spiritual support, particularly when facing the deaths of patients:

> Caring for others who are dying forces us to confront the inevitability of our own death and the death of those we love. How often have

we heard our inner voice say, "This could be me. We're the same age." (p. 33)

Nurses can be supported in stressful work with simple but meaningful acts such as participation in staff support groups or memorial groups where patients are remembered, or by expressions of touch, such as holding the staff member who is experiencing grief. Taylor and Ferszt recommend discussion groups, prayer, and participation in a religious community or formal church. They find that contemplating the cycles of nature (dying and rebirth) is meaningful for nurses.

## ISSUES AND PERSPECTIVES

To practice spirituality within a religious context involves accepting prescribed beliefs concerning God, the meaning and purpose of life, and the nature of an afterlife. All this and more (including what one should *do* in adhering to the faith), can be found within a given church doxology.

Commitment to a specific faith has many advantages for the believer, one being that each individual need not create his interpretation of God and life's meaning from scratch. Of course, the very fact of religious membership may stimulate in some people exactly this sort of intensive inner quest. Spirituality within a religion (instead of unattached) provides a structure for belief as well as satisfying man's basic need to connect to something larger than himself.

A formalized religion supplies a community, a group of like believers, and belonging. Even the Christian scriptures refer to the power achieved when numbers gather together in worship.

### Proselytizing

If the nurse's religion and the patient's differ in significant ways, the nurse must be careful to respect the patient's beliefs and not try to insert her own. It is important to differentiate between the two sets of beliefs. As healer and ordained minister Balistreri (2002) said:

> Usually I start any form of therapy by saying a light prayer. . . . "I invoked the light of the Christ within. I am a clear and perfect healing channel of God's love and light. Light is my guide" . . . I say this out loud so they'll know what I'm doing. I say, "Even if you don't like this, this is for *me*." (p. 103)

Healer and rolfer Bernau-Eigen (2002) also differentiated healer and client beliefs:

> Or the client might say that he needs help. Then I ask, "What is the healing presence for you?" It might be Jesus, Buddha, Allah, or whoever. Then we bring that presence in. The more we can stick with the client's belief system, the better. I keep my beliefs to myself. (p. 85)

In the present era, avid proselytizing is rare. Still, we must ask the question: What is the nurse's path when she is religious, and the patient and his family lack a spiritual belief network? What right, if any, does the nurse have to express to the patient her private views? Or should such views simply be demonstrable, not verbalized, in her behaviors?

What about the opposite case, where the patient and his family are religious, but the nurse is not? Should the nurse hide her skepticism? Should she keep out of it by providing access to accessible spiritual counselors or chaplains? A major religious issue exists, at least for some nurses, where the religious beliefs of the nurse and patient differ.

### Levels of Spiritual/Religious Development

Religion can have different significance even for those who belong to the same group. For some, religion fills an important part in their spiritual lives. For others, faith is more a matter of finding a comfortable social home base, accepting a creed, perhaps with only a superficial understanding of it.

If one grants that there may be various levels of spiritual faith or sophistication, another religious issue emerges: Can spiritual faith or sophistication be a requirement for nurses? What happens when her spiritual care of the patient is limited by the nurse's own level of spiritual development? Spiritual development has seldom been a criterion for nursing entry, graduation, or practice, and religious affiliation is seldom a criterion for education or practice.

If Peck (1993) is right about stages of religious development, a nurse at Stage Two (formal, rule-bound) will be unable to help a patient who has already progressed to Stages Three or Four. Of course calling the priest/minister/rabbi may be of little help either because, as Peck notes, many religious authorities are actually at Stage Two themselves. Recall that Peck identified the following phases of human religious development, Stage One, antisocial, involving an absence of spirituality and unprincipled behavior; Stage Two, formal/institutional, and characterized by submission to the rules; Stage Three, rebellion from unthinking submission, often resulting in doubters, atheists, and agnostics seeking deep truths; and Stage Four, the mystical/communal stage revealing the cohesion beneath the surface of things. (Review chapter 4 for more details.)

The issue here is that neither medical workers nor religious workers are graded on spiritual maturity. But if one grants there may be differences in levels of spiritual maturity, then different nurses may bring different limitations and talents in providing spiritual care to patients.

There is no accounting for spiritual development of nurse, physician, religious leader, or patient. Without some criteria, such as Peck's four stages or Fowler's (1981) seven, the situation defies analysis.

Given the situation, a cynic might argue that it is foolhardy to make spiritual care an element in nursing when (1) it can't be taught, (2) it can't be used as a gatekeeping element in selecting nurses, (3) it fails to take into account the levels of spiritual maturity among practitioners, and (4) it fails to appreciate religious differences.

Yet, ironically, we know that the right nurse at the right place in the right time can bring significant spiritual benefit to the patient. Perhaps the best we can do, given all the difficulties, is to teach nurses that many people have religious and spiritual needs, and that, for them, the needs are very real.

The notion of levels brings us back to the existential fact that the nurse can't be what she isn't. This is not to denigrate the fact that presencing may be important, no matter what the spiritual development or specific religious beliefs of patient or nurse.

## SPIRITUAL BEHAVIORS

Religious and spiritual behaviors of nurses are relatively easy to identify, although their depth may defy classification: prayer, reading spiritual materials, taking to others (patients, families, or nurses) about spiritual matters, worshiping God, and finding purpose and meaning in one's life or that of one's patients.

These behaviors on the part of the nurse are designed to alleviate the stress that accompanies an illness, to enhance the patient's coping abilities, to decrease suffering, to decrease fear in facing death, or, for some nurses in some situations, to help the patient seek salvation. In addition to directing these efforts toward patients, similar tactics may be used with their families. Underlying these activities may lie a compassion for others, a reverence for life, or a religious zeal, among other motivations.

## CREATING A RELIGIOUS NURSING THEORY

If one were interested in creating a new religious theory of nursing, that would certainly be possible. Recall that Longway created such a theory decades ago (see chapters 7, 8, and 9 for details). We could parse Longway's (1970) theory element this way:

*Content:* (1) God as the source of power, (2) illness as stoppage of God's power
*Process:* (1) Patient: falls out of God's redemption and loses power, (2) Nurse: provides energy, motivated by love, for completing the circuit of God
*Context:* (1) God as power, energy
*Goal:* (1) Patient: regain lost God power, (2) Nurse: help patient to lay hold of more energy for himself and thus enable him to advance along the illness–wellness continuum.

There are several key possibilities presented by different authors in this chapter that could be joined to create a religious theory of nursing with the following elements:

*Content:* (1) suffering, (2) dying, (3) finding meaning in life, (4) relating to a higher power
*Process:* (1) accompaniment, (2) finding meaning, (3) relieving suffering
*Context:* (1) creating a healing environment, (2) life as a larger arena than the here and now
*Goal:* (1) salvation (as defined in the given religion), (2) spiritual growth, (3) peace and acceptance.

The specific meanings of these elements would vary from religion to religion, but these elements might provide a basic map for someone interested in creating a religious nursing theory.

### SUMMARY

The relationship between spirituality and organized religion is not a simple one. Not only are there variations among organized religions, but there are differences in specific beliefs among and between nurses, patients, their families, and religious advisers

The nurse needs to be aware of the place of religion in her life and sensitive to religion's importance for her patient. Whether the nurse is qualified to act as religious advisor is not something everyone agrees on. The answer may vary from expert to expert and from nurse to nurse, depending on her spiritual maturity and the specific needs of her patients.

Spirituality did not begin with today's trends. As we noted in chapters 1 and 2, nursing's spiritual origin began in early religions but was particularly enhanced in Christianity, with its focus on service to others. That tradition continues today in many institutions and in many individual nurses.

This chapter focused on spirituality as it is expressed through religion, namely, through a formalized body of religious beliefs to which the patient ascribes, along with membership in a church or other religious organization. The orientation of this chapter was toward the Judeo-Christian religion, with little mention of other groups, nor was there mention of religion misused toward other ends.

For the reader who wonders why so much more content in this book addressed spirituality in the New Age paradigm rather than in traditional religion, the answer is simple: nursing has had few theories grounded in formalized religion. Nurses working within the new paradigm, on the other hand, have published several well-known theories. Indeed, the only internally consistent nursing theory grounded in a religion (and known to this author) is Longway's (1970) Seventh Day Adventist theory. Meux and Rooda (1995) presented a theory that cast religion as a cultural component, but the model was ultimately culture driven rather than grounded totally in religion.

As with Meux and Rooda, nurses do create theories with an appreciation of respective religions. But aspects of formalized religions seldom appear as major theory components. It may well be that this era will be the one in which a full-fledged religion-based nursing theory will be formulated. Several authors have bitten off chunks that may evolve into full theories. Donley (1991), for example, offered an excellent analysis of the concept of *suffering* within a religious context. Similarly, Roberts and Whall's (1996) variable, *serenity*, (discussed in chapter 11) could be adopted in either a new paradigm or a religious theory

In order for a religious theory of nursing to arise, it will be necessary to delve into the great divide between science and religion. As Keller (1988) said concerning Christianity:

> [we] must not squeeze the Bible into the Procrustean bed of our demands for "historical truth" and "scientific objectivity" which are themselves sufficiently problematical. It is, or rather, it was an historical work, but not such as we understand the term. It is the account of a people and its god, whose powers his worshippers came to know in the course of history. The Bible does not attempt to be a neutral, objective account of the events it relates. It is far too committed for that, much too rooted in its own times. (p. 437)

Religion in present nursing care is most often present as context, providing an underlying valuing environment within which nursing is given and received.

## REFERENCES

Armstrong, K. (1993). *A history of God.* New York: Ballantine Books.

Baer, E. D, Fagin, C. M., & Gordon, S. (Eds.). (1996). *Abandonment of the patient: The impact of profit-driven health care on the public.* New York: Springer.

Balistreri, K. (2002). Interview. In B. Barnum, *The new healers: Minds and hands in complementary medicine* (pp. 97–107). Long Branch, NJ: Vista.

Bernau-Eigen, M. (2002). Interview. In B. Barnum, *The new healers: Minds and hands in complementary medicine* (pp. 72–87). Long Branch, NJ: Vista.

Borchert, B. (1994). *Mysticism: Its history and challenge.* York Beach, ME: Samuel Weiser.

Cimino, J. E. (1984 May 20). *Non-abandonment: Physicians and nurses as allies.* Unpublished convocation address, School of Medicine, State University at Stony Brook, New York.

Deikman, A. J. (1972). Deautomatization and the mystic experience. In C. T. Tart (Ed.), *Altered states of consciousness* (3rd ed., pp. 34–57). San Francisco: Harper SanFrancisco.

Donley, R., Sr. (1991). Spiritual dimensions of health care: Nursing's mission. *Nursing & Health Care, 12*(4), 178–183.

Fowler, J. (1981). *Stages of faith.* New York: HarperCollins.

George, L. (1995). *Alternative realities: The paranormal, the mystic and the transcendent in human experience.* New York: FactsOnFile.

Hillman, J. (1996). *The soul's code: In search of character and calling.* New York: Warner Books.

Johnson, R. A. (1986). *Inner work: Using dreams and active imagination for personal growth.* San Francisco: Harper SanFrancisco.

Keller, W. (1988). *The Bible as history.* New York: Bantam Books.

Kerfoot, K. (1995) Today's patient care unit manager: Keeping spirituality in managed care: The nurse manager's challenge. *Nursing Economic$, 13*(1), 49–51.

Krieger, D. (1981). *Foundations for holistic health nursing practices: The renaissance nurse.* Philadelphia: J. B. Lippincott.

Longway, I. (1970, February/March). Toward a philosophy of nursing. *Journal of Adventist Education, 32*(3), 20–27.

Matthews, D. (1997). Faith and medicine: Reconciling the twin traditions of healing. *Mind/Body Medicine, 2*(1), 3–6.

Maupin, E. W. (1972). On meditation. In C. T. Tart (Ed.), *Altered states of consciousness* (3rd ed., pp. 217–240). San Francisco: HarperSanFrancisco.

McKivergin, M. (2000). The nurse as an instrument of healing. In B. M. Dossey, L. Keegan, & C. E. Guzzetta (Eds.), *Holistic nursing: A handbook for practice* (3rd ed., pp. 207–227). Gaithersburg, MD: Aspen.

Meux, L., & Rooda, L. A. (1995, June) The development of a model for delivery of religio-specific nursing care. *Journal of Holistic Nursing, 13*(2), 132–141.

Moore, T. (1994). *Care of the soul*. New York: Harper Perennial.

Peck, M. S. (1993). *Further along the road less traveled: The unending journey toward spiritual growth*. New York: Simon & Schuster.

Roberts, K. T., & Whall, A. (1996, Winter). Serenity as a goal for nursing practices. *Image, 28*(4), 359–364.

Spector, R. E. (1996). *Cultural diversity in health & illness* (4th ed.). Stamford, CT: Apppleton & Lange.

Taylor, P. B., & Ferszt, G. G. (1990). Spiritual healing. *Holistic Nursing Practice, 4*(4), 32–38.

Taylor, R., & Watson, J. (1989). *They shall not hurt: Human suffering and human caring*. Boulder, CO: Colorado Associated University Press.

Thich Nhat Hanh (1998). *The heart of Buddha's teaching*. New York: Broadway Books.

# PART VI

## Spirituality and Ethics

The renewed interest in spirituality often is linked, not to the new paradigm, but simply to the increasing number and complexity of problems in today's society. Specifically, in health care, the renewed interest in spirituality is connected to the increasing puzzles and perplexities in ethics, which in turn relate to administrative regulations and legal codes. The expanding interest in ethics arose when new circumstances, especially modern technology, created unique quandaries for which there were no prescribed rules of conduct. Cloning possibilities and use of embryonic tissue from aborted fetuses are examples of developing realities for which the rules are not yet stable.

Ethics is the study of what is right and wrong, good and bad, or correct action. A society usually reflects these dominant values in its laws, but the laws tend to lag behind the social changes. Both the values and the laws are constantly in flux as society evolves.

Part VI examines some of the links between spirituality and ethics without attempting in any way to provide a comprehensive review of ethics. Indeed, ethics and medical ethics are extensive domains. The following two chapters give only the briefest indication of the interface between spirituality and ethics. The reader wishing a basic text in ethics as it applies to nursing might select Bandman and Bandman (2001).

Although spirituality, like ethics, relates to human values, it is more a question of what makes the human spirit soar, what links man to higher powers, however defined. Spirituality does not set out to determine codes of behavior, although spiritual beliefs may drastically affect the behaviors chosen by the believer.

Ethics (or morality), has more to do with regulating people and their relationships with each other than with the relationship between a person and God. Because ethics deals with relationships among people, it is not surprising to find it intertwined with legal considerations. Rules for the conduct of people evolve from the generally accepted ethical values of a given nation in a given era.

Chapter 13 examines some trends in medical ethics in the United States, more specifically, the ethical problems facing nurses. Chapter 14 relates moral problems to various philosophies of ethics. Sources of moral decision making are differentiated and compared. The chief message is that all sorts of people consider themselves ethical yet reach quite different conclusions.

Because all actions can be interpreted from a position of ethics, the nurse cannot avoid making decisions in the domain of right and wrong, good and bad. Even the nurse who always follows the rules, that is, administrative dictates, is making ethical decisions every time he or she decides to let the rules make the decisions.

Because ethics is the study of right and wrong, it is closely associated with spirituality, a concept about the greatest source of meaning. One could say that one's notions of spirituality serve as a context in which ethical decisions are made. Certainly one's spiritual beliefs determine which ethical structures are acceptable and which are not.

### REFERENCE

Bandman, E. L., & Bandman, B. (2001). *Nursing ethics through the life span* (4th ed.). Norwalk, CT: Appleton & Lange.

# Chapter 13

## Spirituality and Ethics: A Contrast in Forms

**M**oral quandaries comprise the domain of ethical inquiry; hence, most discussions of ethics focus on decision making. In contrast, spirituality is more often a matter of context than of decision making. Ethics offers no sense of lifting the human spirit upward; it often comes with a sense of burden and always a sense of duty. Spirituality and ethics both have to do with what is right and wrong, but they connote different images, different ways of handling oneself in the world.

Discussions of ethics often concern problems and vulnerabilities—situations in which the nurse might possibly do the wrong thing. Spirituality, on the other hand, relates to the joyous experiences of soul growth and connection with a higher good. We might call spirituality the larger term, ethics the more limited and practical one. Medical ethics seeks to determine how to manage health-related problems when people disagree over the right action.

Three circumstances predominate in creating today's ethical complexities: (1) new technologies, (2) issues of resource scarcity, and (3) increasing sensitivity to human rights.

### NEW TECHNOLOGIES

New technology spurs ethical issues with virtually every major advancement. For example, the ability to impregnate older women, some in their sixties, raises the issue of whether it is ethical to give birth to a child who is likely to be orphaned at an early age. The ability to implant donor eggs in women no longer young enough to be fertile reflects the interplay of law, ethics, and social structures. The technology is useful in a society where many career women delay beginning childbearing. Further, the United States has an influx of women from other countries where post-menopausal impregnation is illegal, seeking the technology here.

Cloning is perhaps the greatest change on the immediate horizon (and therefore the greatest potential for ethical debate). The technological capability of cloning humans will be reached soon, possibly before this book is in the reader's hands. And if it is possible, it is inevitable that someone will do it. One issue here is whether it is right (or wrong) to reproduce an exact duplicate of a human being. Here we might note an interlink of ethics and spirituality. Many spiritual positions would hold that an exact duplicate is not produced, that an identical body would be inhabited by a different soul. Indeed, the existence of identical twins already presents such a situation. We even have some situations where mothers fertilized at different times by in vitro frozen embryos have given birth to identical twins years apart. Few "spiritual" viewpoints would see the clone as identical to the original person, but some scientific viewpoints might take that position.

A more critical issue involves the old "spare parts" argument, with fears of human clones being used as depositories of spare parts for the "originals," rather than achieving full human rights. In our culture, at least at present, that fear seems far-fetched. Indeed, this concept has already been applied in several cases where parents elected to birth a child with hopes that it would be a donor match for transplants needed by another child in the family.

Another recent source of ethical problems is the use of stem cells from aborted fetuses. The pro arguments include the hope that they may be invaluable in curing serious diseases. The con side deals with the notion of abortion and the fear that some fetuses would be created just for medical use. Issues of just when fetal cells are considered a human being enter into this debate. A spiritual link here might involve notions of human life, for example, when does a soul enter the body?

In new circumstances such as these, much of what the nurse does is simply providing information and clarity for persons at large. For example, a nurse may be asked to explain cloning. Explanations, however, are often given, for good or ill, in ways that advance personal ethical stances.

Further along the life chain, serious moral quandaries are raised in saving immature infants who may, consequently, live with numerous physical and mental disabilities. The issue here is quality of life versus life at any price. Ethical positions vary on how this question is answered, as do spiritual perceptions on living and dying.

On the other edge of life, one finds additional ethical questions concerning quality of life. When quality is compromised, can we speed up death by acts of omission? Acts of commission? What about the preferences of the person? Are we to accept elected suicide? One thinks, for example, of the Hemlock

Society, named in recognition of Socrates' death; the Society actually teaches people how to commit suicide. In extreme cases, selected death may deal with euthanasia. Is there ever a case when the quality of life is so poor that the society (or others than the person involved ) have the right to decide on euthanasia? Rice, Beck, and Stevenson (1997) link such ethical issues to the increasing number of cognitively impaired elders in our society, a problem itself created by medical technology that prolongs life.

Patients and their families are now demanding their rights in such decision-making processes. Issues that once were settled by an authoritarian physician have become negotiations in which many persons have a stake and in which life-at-any-cost is seldom seen as the right answer.

The ethical dilemma is complicated by the legal issue, that is, the vulnerability of those who take measures to stop or prevent life-preserving therapy. At least four levels of involvement in terminating a life exist for the professional: (1) stopping treatments that prolong life, (2) giving treatments that relieve symptoms but may cause death as a side effect, (3) assisting in suicide, and (4) performing euthanasia. At the moment many individuals, as well as the society as a whole, struggle with these differences. People have different opinions concerning which of these actions, and under what conditions, are ethical. Nurses, obviously, have different levels of comfort with these options, given their own ethical codes.

At the final boundary, our ability to prolong the life of the body creates another set of ethical problems: What does it mean to be alive? When does death occur? When may a body be harvested for organs? What are the dangers of excessive zeal versus delay that may damage organs?

Many spiritual beliefs include a notion of an afterlife, and for people holding these beliefs, the idea of death is less threatening than it is to many who hold the scientific paradigm. What is "ethical," then, can change depending on one's beliefs concerning an afterlife.

Over time, the situations that raise ethical questions tend to be solved, normalized, often legalized, and then raise few questions. Consider, for example, the ethical furor that arose concerning the first "test tube" baby. Now that situation is so routine that virtually no one thinks of in vitro fertilization as an ethical problem.

Technology keeps creating novel situations for which normative patterns of right and wrong have yet to be settled. Circumstances such as these confound people and institutions. Most want to do the right thing, but determining what is right can be fraught with dangers, not to mention the threat of legal action. More and more people settle ethical problems by way of the courts, not because they lack opinions as to the best course, not even because they disagree on the best course, but because a court decision leaves everyone less vulnerable to prosecution.

Ethics is fraught with the need for decision making, rule setting, and keeping of obligations. Ethical positions, when contended at court, lead to legal dictates. Legal precedents mount, creating paths of public policy. Spirituality, in contrast, tends not to be a public thing, but a private thing. Yet growing spiritual trends can eventually have an influence on what is or is not considered an ethical problem.

There are many links between ethics and spirituality. Watson (1999) captures one difference in the following:

> A nurse may perform actions toward a patient out of a sense of duty or moral obligation, and would be an ethical nurse. Yet it may be false to say he or she cared about the patient. The value of human care and caring involves a higher sense of spirit of self. (p. 31)

## RESOURCE SCARCITY

Ethical issues arise when there are not enough needed supplies/therapies to go around. Sometimes that lack is based in economics. New technologies and new health care products have increased the range of health care options, yet the cost of these innovations often exceeds the ability of the society to pay for them. Society must decide which options will be developed and which will not, as well as who will receive their benefit when the technology is in scarce supply.

Other times, the scarcity may be traced to nontechnological sources, for example the scarcity of body organs for transplant. The effects are the same, whatever the source of the scarcity. In either case, the issue becomes one of access, namely, who will receive the needed therapy? Who will not, and for what reason? Attempts to set rationales for distribution of scarce resources have always been fraught with problems in this nation. And the disagreements are easy to understand: people put different values on different criteria.

Take a simple case where there is one liver and two potential recipients. The surgeon might prefer to transplant to the patient who is in better physical status because his chances of survival are better. Others on the staff might argue for the sicker patient on the theory that it is his last opportunity. Others might wish to select the patient on the basis of productive years left, while others might want to use prior life style as a selection factor. These kinds of values don't contrast a wrong and a right against each other; instead, they force a choice between various goods.

Interestingly, much of the literature written by nurses gives cases where a nurse fights for his or her patient to receive a scarce resource. Usually the only ethical consideration is simply that the particular person was the nurse's patient. This brings the issue of advocacy into the realm of ethics. Advocacy for "my patient" versus others simply because of the personal association is debatable on ethical terms. Hamric (2000) gives a good analysis of patient advocacy as a nursing role from an ethics position.

One major ethical problem is how to resolve the tension between a continuously developing science whose technology prolongs and enhances life versus the costs to society. Notice that this conflict occurs only when one accepts two normative sets of values simultaneously: (1) the medical ideology that prolonged or enhanced life is of prime value, and (2) the social-economic preference to place a limit on the fiscal investment in the health of people. In other words, there is a limit to the funds directed into the nation's health research and development, and the limit is insufficient for all the desirable goals that might be achieved.

There is also the legitimate problem of the few versus the many. Drug companies are forced to deal with this pressure, for example, when they determine to research common diseases instead of orphan diseases, that is, diseases that affect a small percentage of the population. It is easy for others to castigate the drug companies for ignoring the problems of the few because of the small projected financial payoff compared to the costs of research and development for these esoteric conditions. Yet drug company officials could argue that their aim was beneficent: to help more people rather than fewer people. And, as we see all the time, the visibility of one affected celebrity can change which diseases receive attention and which do not.

The issue of scarcity involves the issue of equity. Most reasonable people would agree that health care should be distributed equitably, yet what constitutes equity is not so simple. One party's equity is another's deprivation.

What about the inequity when parents from different social strata, with different means, compete for a scarce resource, for example, a liver for a dying child? What about the rights of a financially stressed surrogate mother versus the rights of the wealthy contracting father? What about those institutions that seek to enhance their shaky financial bases by creating more expensive units for patients who can afford those special extras? It is apparent that the issues quickly escape the medical category to flow over into larger questions of social justice.

The cases and causes are numerous, but in each example one asks: Who decides? Who pays? Who has rights? Who has obligations? What is justice? The problem in making most of these decisions is that, once again, the choices do not involve choosing between right and wrong, good and bad; instead they involve choosing between opposing goods.

Although she was only addressing end-of-life decisions, Tilden (1999) gives three ethics principles that can serve as criteria in almost any ethical choice: autonomy, beneficence, and justice. Autonomy concerns preserving patient decision making, beneficence weighs costs and benefits of the decision, and justice views the decision from a societal viewpoint.

Notice that when one discusses morality in terms of rights, justice, and equity, the argument usually hinges on the older world-view. In a New Age paradigm, rights and equity often dissolve into broad perspectives, possibly involving reincarnation and ultimate soul growth. A nurse operating in this paradigm may feel that there is not adequate knowledge to make any judgments concerning what is fair or equitable. Her principles arise from other sources. A nurse holding a New Age ideology might find the problem of scarcity beside the point. She might argue that prolonging or enhancing life is not itself an important goal. She might hold that solving these problems could obstruct the soul development of persons who have elected to experience lives cut short at a young age or lives lived in difficult situations. Indeed, she might consider the markers of life, death, and comfort to be inconsequential in the longer view of a soul's development over various lifetimes.

The point to be made here is that ethics are very much tied to a nurse's world-view. One's accepted world paradigm will ultimately dictate which nursing theories and which ethical theories will appeal. In the past era, when most nurses in this culture shared the same world view, almost everyone accepted that disease was bad and should be alleviated in every form, and that the health of everyone should be improved until we reached the place of ideal health care for everybody at all times. Within this framework, even different ethical positions could be discussed from a common beginning point. That is no longer the case in nursing.

## NEW SENSITIVITY TO HUMAN RIGHTS

Every state in the Union is dealing with new laws concerning human rights. Among medical rights, none is more pervasive than issues concerning the quality of life. Even under the older normative ideology, changes were coming about in ethical values in relation to this issue. Quality of life is the first value to confront head-on the medical assumption that the preservation of life is always to be desired.

Women's health rights also have emerged as ethical issues. In the past, far too often only men have been used as research subjects. This tactic has caused differences in health response between the sexes to be ignored. Often treatments best for men have later been determined not to be best for women. Studies of heart attack victims were prominent in this sort of study flaw, and now efforts are underway to include women as subjects in most major research studies.

Ethics problems even include consideration of unequal treatment of sexes with the same diagnoses. See, for example, Hoffman and Tarzian (2001), who found differences in treatment of pain. As they report, "Women, it seems, have to 'prove' that they are as sick as men in order to receive the same level of pain treatment." Obviously, people are being sensitized to pain treatment inequities because of new Joint Commission on Accreditation of Healthcare Organization's (JCAHO) standards for pain management. However, the fact remains that unequal treatment reflects a gender bias that is clearly unethical.

We now see a growing global awareness concerning such things as women's rights to health and education, cessation of cultural mutilation of women's bodies, and other human rights that often involve health issues. Distribution of drugs for AIDS in third-world countries is another example of global concern.

## INSTITUTIONAL ETHICS

Institutions of health care, by their very nature, draw and create ethical quandaries. Ethical issues arise for the nurse in several ways: (1) being caught between physician demands and actions they believe to be right for the patient, (2) peer pressures on a care unit, and (3) institutional policies that ignore patients' rights or desires. Nurses often feel pressured to yield to physician, peer, or organizational power and status. Hamric (2001) captures these issues in an article aptly titled, "Reflections on Being in the Middle."

Additionally, some nurses fear that their organizations would not support them for ethical stands taken on disputable issues. In some circumstances, nurses feel powerless to implement the decisions that they feel to be morally right.

Because no individual action is likely to be supported as ethical by every player in a case, what matters from an institutional viewpoint is that no participant be forced to take part in an action offensive to his or her particular ethical stance. This protection of the individual nurse (and other participants) is an organizational obligation.

In regular nursing practice, issues having ethical implications surface with regularity. They include but are not limited to: do-not-resuscitate practices; management for suspected child, wife, or elder abuse; patients' rights to informed consent, privacy, and confidentiality; the patient's right to die; reproductive rights; and quality of life issues.

Most institutions deal with ethical problems through an ethics committee that decides on the best action in ambiguous cases. These committees prevent arbitrary and premature decision making in complex cases. Even on an ethics committee, however, there may be honest moral disagreements. The use of deliberative committee decision making, however, provides some legal protection. Legal judgments may be sought by the institution in particularly complex cases.

An institutional review board provides another clearing house for ethical problems—those that arise in all research endeavors using patients as subjects. Even though a review board may be composed of people holding different beliefs, there is merit to joint deliberation. The quality of decision making certainly is improved by a thoughtful process.

## WHO DECIDES?

Probably the greatest change in recent years has been the growing involvement of people in their own health care decisions. The patient (or his family as surrogate) is now expected to participate in full and informed decision making regarding his condition, prognosis, and treatment.

The American Nurses' Association's (2001) *Code for Nurses* provides guidelines concerning nurses' obligations to patients, colleagues, and the larger society. It does not, except in the broadest of terms, address specific ethical issues. It cannot tell the nurse what to do in particular situations. The code is a useful guide, but ethical decisions still need to be puzzled out individually in each case. The code falls prey to the flaws of any document that attempts to use generalized rules of behavior to dictate concrete, specific actions.

## SUMMARY

Unlike the broad spiritual focus, the ethical focus tends to be on problems. Present ethical problems arise from many sources, including situations created by new technology, resource scarcity, and new sensitivities to human rights. This chapter aims only at sensitizing the reader to ethical problems and differentiating ethics from spirituality.

While both ethics and spirituality involve what is right and wrong, their images differ. Ethics focuses on rights and duties, on equity and justice, often with a rule orientation. Ethics calls forth an image of a code of acceptable behavior. Spirituality, on the other hand, evokes an image of life lived and experienced in light of certain beliefs and meanings given to life and higher levels of existence. At present both ethics and spirituality are important in nursing. While not at odds with each other, they represent different perspectives on underlying moral concerns.

## REFERENCES

American Nurses' Association (2001). *Code for nurses with interpretive statement.* Washington DC: Author.

Hamric, A. B. (2000, May/June). What is happening to advocacy? *Nursing Outlook, 48*(3), 103–104.

Hamric, A. B. (2001, November/December). Reflections on being in the middle. *Nursing Outlook, 49*(6), 254–257.

Hoffman, D. E., & Tarzian, A. J. (2001, Spring). The girl who cried pain: A bias against women in the treatment of pain. Internet version of *American Journal of Law and Medicine, 29*(1), http://www.aslme.org/pub-jlme/exec-sum-29.1html

Rice, V. H., Beck, C., & Stevenson, J. S. (1997, January/February). Ethical issues relative to autonomy and personal control in independent and cognitively impaired elders. *Nursing Outlook, 45*(1), 27–34.

Tilden, V. (1999, July/August). Ethics perspectives on end-of-life care. *Nursing Outlook, 47*(4), 162–167.

Watson, J. (1999). *Nursing: Human science and human care: A theory of nursing.* Boston: Jones and Bartlett.

# Chapter 14

## Ethics and Philosophy

As we said in chapter 13, when one turns from spirituality to ethics (at least as the notion appears in nursing), there is a radical shift in orientation. This chapter looks at ethics as a distinct field of philosophic inquiry.

### A PHILOSOPHICAL OVERVIEW OF ETHICS

In addition to the practical differences between traditional ethics and emerging notions of spirituality, there are disparities among the philosophic approaches used in the systematic study of ethics. These differences can be discussed in a branching decision tree (see Figure 14.1).

The first differentiation is between philosophies of *determinism* and human *freedom*. In determinism, all things happen in terms of antecedents. If one knew what had happened in the past, one could predict the present action of any person. In this belief system, there is no such thing as free will; one's choices are determined by what happened earlier. Consequently, in this system it is a misnomer to use the term ethics. If all choices are the inevitable result of earlier events, then one cannot be morally accountable for his or her acts.

To allow for ethics, there first must be some freedom of choice; one must be able to choose right over wrong—or wrong over right for that matter. Hence the rest of our branching philosophies all fall within the concept of human freedom.

Even among theories that espouse freedom of choice (free will), there are alternate positions: in one formulation, *ethical choice* exists; in the other, *moral skepticism* holds forth. Moral skepticism claims that, while people are free to choose, their choices are not influenced by ethics. Moral choice is illusory in

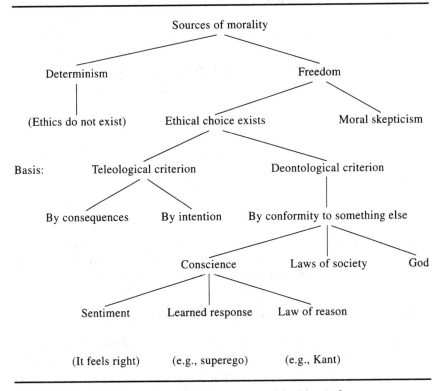

**FIGURE 14.1** Why good people disagree on ethical issues?

moral skepticism; ethics is an empty word. People choose all right, but not on the basis of what is good or bad. They choose for other reasons, for example, self-interest. If an ethical position is offered, it is simply a rationalization.

Among the positions that support the existence of *ethical choice*, there is yet another differentiation, depending on the *way* something is known to be ethical. Here there are two possible answers, *teleologic* or *deontologic*.

Teleology refers to the outcome, result, or goal. Teleological systems assert that people make choices based on what will happen, given their decisions. This assumes that one has some capacity to predict results of given actions. Within teleological systems, we find yet another branching point. Suppose a man, using a teleological perspective, decided to kill his dying wife to save her pain. Suppose, also, that a week later a cure was found for her disease. Some ethicists would judge his act ethical according to its *intentions*. It was ethical because, given what the man knew, he intended the best for her.

Another ethicist might judge the act according to its actual *consequences*. These ethicists would judge the man's act unethical because he destroyed a woman who might have recovered had he not killed her.

Notice that the very same act was ethical when evaluated in one system and unethical when viewed from the another. Yet both of these systems judge the ethics of an act from its outcome.

The *deontological* position does not judge an act by its outcome. Neither the person's intentions nor the act's consequences are considered. Instead, deontology judges an act to be ethical based on its conformity with something else. The something else, as you might suspect, varies from philosophy to philosophy, giving us other branching points. Three common options are: (1) the *laws* of the society, (2) *God* (or His revealed word, however conceptualized), or (3) one's *conscience*.

Let us look at just one of these options, conscience, to illustrate the complexity. Assume the rule of ethics is, "Let your conscience be your guide." Quickly a problem arises, namely that different consciences dictate different acts. Just look at the abortion rights issue and proponents on both sides of that issue. Each side is convinced that its conscience is absolutely correct.

Further, there are many different interpretations of conscience. Some see it is a *learned response*. One might place Freud's internalization of the super-ego in this category. In this case, a conscience is formed by internalizing the parent. What the parent teaches as good or bad will form the conscience in this perspective. We might look at the thoroughly indoctrinated suicide bomber here. He has been taught to believe that his killing act is a moral martyrdom.

A second interpretation of conscience might be that it is the *law of reason*. Here one might refer to logical rules like Kant's categorical imperative (1986). Kant said that one must act in such a way that the rest of humankind could perform the very same act. For example, if I were considering performing euthanasia on a patient who was not in a condition to request it, I would have to think through what would happen if every other person in the world also committed euthanasia as they saw fit. This picture would act as a check on my behavior, because, obviously, I would not trust the rest of mankind to all do this same act.

Another interpretation finds that conscience rests in *sentiment*. The "inner voice" theory represents this view: Do whatever feels right, follow your heart. Of course, those inner voices can be tricky. If one responds to an inner voice, it is still possible to ask how that inner voice makes its decisions. Does it intuit that certain *rules* are good? In this case sentiment might follow rules like Never tell a lie. Don't commit murder. Or does the sentiment function to judge each act separately? In the latter view, it might be right to murder in one case (when the axe murderer is attacking one's children), but not in another case.

This brief presentation of the field of ethics highlights the complexities that arise when one attempts to analyze the basis for ethical decision making. People of good will, all of whom identify themselves as moral, may disagree in good faith.

## COMPARING PERSPECTIVES

In light of these different bases for ethics, one might analyze the ongoing ethical dispute between the perspectives of Kohlberg and Gilligan on moral development. Nurses are typically inclined to resist Kohlberg's theories because the studies of nurses (and women) using this model usually classify them as morally immature.

Kohlberg's (1981) classification for moral development used a rule-bound, *deontological* system, leaning heavily on concepts of justice and equity. The premise for Kohlberg's system was challenged by Gilligan (1982), who claimed that female morality was not immature but derived from personal relationships rather than abstract concepts. In essence, Gilligan asserted that women's ethics are more commonly *teleological*.

Neither party, of course, used these ethical categories in discussing their systems. Notice that if one takes a given position as absolute, any other system, when measured according to that given position, will be found wanting. Hence, anyone who functions on a teleological system is bound to test poorly if the scale assumes that a deontological position is correct.

## ETHICS AND THE PHILOSOPHY OF MAN

What is valued in a society depends not only on one's philosophic stance on ethics, but on how the human being himself is viewed. One's ethical position, in other words, may be influenced by one's conception of the human being. The following list gives some different ways in which the person may be conceptualized:

The human being

1. is made in the image of God, and this accounts for his value above all other creations. Indeed, the rest of the world was created for his use.
2. is just another animal; his supremacy is his anthropomorphic view of himself. He is differentiated by his advanced ability to use tools, but there is no reason this trait is inherently better than the cat's ability to run faster or the fish's ability to withdraw oxygen from water.
3. is differentiated from other animals by his rationality; he is the only animal capable of abstract thought. He is supreme by virtue of his mind.

4. is differentiated from other animals because he asks the question, "What is man?" He is the only animal who questions his own existence and nature. What makes him different is his ability for introspective, reflexive thoughts.

5. does not exist in the usual sense of the word. What exists is what is perceived. Therefore only the mind has a real, separate existence; all other things such as animals, earth, and a person's body exist only insofar as they are conceived to exist by the mind.

6. is a bundle of sense perceptions. He continually changes as his perceptions change. The sense of a single continuous "me" is an illusion; there is no durable, unchanging part of the human being. He is a flux of changing sense perceptions.

7. is the only animal endowed with a soul. He is the animal who persists through time, that is, his soul continues to exist when his earthly body and mind perish.

8. is a unity, a single substance. Perceived differences between body and mind are illusory. Mental and physical phenomena represent different expressions of the same substance. When this substance loses its vitality, there is no existence for a person beyond his temporal being.

9. is an integral experience, a lived-body. He cannot be explained by reference to selected parts of his being, for parts cannot explain the whole. Nor can he be explained by psychic or physiologic states, because these are static states, a standing still that is not consistent with the continual change experienced by man. Man is a unified and ongoing lived experience.

10. is a holoscopic component of God, participating with other humans and the rest of creation to form the totality of God or Tao. Although partial and differentiated, he reflects the undifferentiated, unitary nature of Being.

11. is one of many ensouled carbon-based species that live in the universe. The only ensouled land animal on the planet Earth, he enters a life of the spirit, an alternate simultaneous reality, upon release from the carbon-based body by death.

One's philosophic belief about man has a direct effect on judgments concerning ethics. For example, murder would be a horrendous crime for the person holding the view that a person is a temporal being whose only existence is in the here and now. Someone holding a view that this present life is only one phase of existence, maybe a difficult one at that, might consider murder less significant.

## SUMMARY

Even the ethics of the older world paradigm has plenty of room for disagreement. The different schools of ethics, with their varied bases, reveal the reasons for this. Further, one's philosophical view of man and his relation to higher meaning adds another dimension that may influence one's interpretation of morality.

Older ethical perspectives and the new spiritualism often seem to arise out of different conceptions of the world. They appear different for valid reasons. What they share is a focus on values and the need to negotiate between personal beliefs and societal norms.

Whatever bases are used for decision making, the problem for the health professional is that he or she is often placed in an environment where a choice and an action cannot be avoided. Often a decision not to act, is itself a decision. In these circumstances, the nurse should make choices based on some knowledge of ethical decision making rather than in a vacuum.

## REFERENCES

Gilligan, C. (1982). *In a different voice: Psychological theory and women's development*. Cambridge, MA: Harvard University Press.

Kant, I. (1986). Foundations of the metaphysics of morals. In E. Behler (Ed.), *Immanuel Kant: Philosophical writings* (pp. 52–125). New York: Continuum.

Kohlberg, L. (1981). *The meaning and measurement of moral development*. Worcester, MA: Clark University Press.

# Index

**A**
afterlife
　and hypnotic regression, 42
　and near-death experiences, 84, 99–102
　and out-of-body exploration, 42
　and pre-death encounters, 98–99
altered states of consciousness
　and alternative medicine, 6
　in Greek practices, 25
　investigations in, 41–45
　in self-improvement programs, 12–13
alternative medicine therapies
　and altered states of consciousness, 6
　changed perception of, 6
　and changing beliefs, 7
　research in, 6
aura, 131

**B**
bioenergetics
　and healing, 131–133
　in spiritual therapeutics, 152–156
　therapeutic touch, 153–156
body work
　definition of, 115
　value and task clashes, 124–127
　as viewed in nursing theories, 121–123
brain
　brain structures and spirituality, 80–82
　and mystic visions, 82–84
　and reality of spiritual experience,
　　86–87, 88–91
　and spirituality, 79–91

**C**
chakras, 131

channeling, 47–48
cosmic consciousness, and meditation, 85

**D**
death and dying
　beliefs concerning, 96–97
　and hospice movement, 97
　pre-death encounters, 98–99
developmental theories
　and challenges for the nurse, 66, 115
　Erikson, 51–53
　humanistic, 57–59
　Maslow, 53–57
　and psychological schools, 64
　spirituality in, 51–66
　transcendent, 59–64
　transpersonal levels in, 61

**E**
ethics
　and American Nurses' Association
　　guidelines, 192
　and cloning, 186
　and human rights, 190–191
　institutional ethics, 191–192
　and the legal system, 187–188
　in New Age paradigm, 190
　and new technologies, 185–188
　philosophical overview of, 195–198
　and quality of life, 186–187, 190
　and resource scarcity, 188–190
　and spirituality, 185–192
　and terminating life, 186–187
　and theories of moral development,
　　198
　and use of stem cells, 186

ethics *(continued)*
    and view of human being, 198–199
    and women's health rights, 190–191

**F**
faith, helping the patient maintain, 172

**G**
Greek practices
    goddesses associated with nursing, 26
    mystery schools, 24–25
    seers in, 25

**H**
healing
    bioenergetic healing, 131–133
    imagination and intention, 135–136
    modalities, 130–135
    in new paradigm, 130–134
    nurse versus non-nurse healers,
        136–137
    prayer, 134–135
    religious healing, 134–135
    sound therapy, 133–134
    versus curing, 129–130
    *See also* spiritual therapeutics
holistic health centers, 16
holistic nursing, 10
hospice, 16, 97
hypnotic regression
    and afterlife, 42
    and memories of God and creation, 44
    research on, 41–45
    and spiritual therapeutics, 145

**I**
illness
    beliefs concerning, 94–95
    giving meaning to, 170–171
    relation of self to, 95–96

**M**
Maslow's model
    Being cognition, 56–57
    Being values, 54, 55

and Gowan, 60–61
    peak experiences, 54
    self-actualization, 55–56
    transcendence, 55–56
medieval times
    deaconess movement in, 28–29
    hospitals in, 27–28
    and Knights Hospitallers, 28
    nurses in, 28–29
meditation
    brain research on, 85–86
    and religious contemplation, 167
    in spiritual therapeutics, 150–151
mystic visions
    and brain structure, 82–84

**N**
near-death experiences
    and afterlife, 84
    the bad NDE, 100–102
    the good NDE, 99–100
    and nurse responsibilities, 100
    research into, 99–102
New Age spirituality
    elements of, 7
    and nursing theory, 124–127
    and self-improvement programs, 12–13
new care delivery models
    adding new practices, 13–14
    creating new organizing patterns,
        15–16
    incidental effects, 17
    modifying the context, 14–15
    and spirituality, 13–17
new paradigm
    and changes in nursing, 8–11
    nursing theories in, 113–128
    and pragmatism, 6–8
    and scientific world-view, 5–6, 9
    versus old paradigm, 5–11
Nightingale
    and mysticism, 30–31
    and spirituality, 29–32
nursing education, spirituality in, 9–11
nursing history

druids, 26–27
early Roman times, 27
Greek practices, 24–26
medieval times, 27–29
modern linkages, 32–33
Nightingale, 29–32
shamanism, 21–24
nursing theories
in new paradigm, 113–128
and the nursing process, 121–123
religious nursing theory, 178, 179–180
role of values in, 107
and the self, 120
spirituality as a component of,
107–110
value and task clashes, 124–127
and view of disease, 121

**O**
out-of-body exploration
and afterlife, 42
research on, 41–45

**P**
paradigm, *See* new paradigm
parish nursing, 15–16
philosophy
epistemology, 40
logical positivism and nursing, 41
metaphysics, 40
and modern physics, 40
and spirituality, 39–45
physics
and Eastern religious traditions, 37
and mysticism, 41
Newtonian, 37–38
and objectivity, 38–39
quantum mechanics, 38
and spirituality, 37–39
pragmatism, and new paradigm, 6
prayer
in healing, 134–135
studies on the efficacy of, 165–166
in traditional spiritual therapeutics,
165–166

psychology
changes in, 45
and spirituality, 45–47
*See also* transpersonal psychology
psychosomatic healing, 7
psychotherapy and spirituality
alcoholism, 75
multiple personality, 74–75
possession, 73–74

**R**
religion
issues and perspectives, 175–177
and levels of spiritual/religious
development, 176–177
and the nurse, 174–175
and proselytizing, 175–176
religious counselors, 173
religious nursing theory, 178, 179–180
as source of strength, 163–164
and spiritual therapeutics, 163–180
religious therapies
giving meaning to illness and
suffering, 170–171
helping the patient maintain faith, 172
and New Age therapies, 173–174
prayer, 165–166
presencing, 166–167
religious contemplation, 167–169
ritual, 169–170
repatterning, 144–145

**S**
scientific world-view
impact on patient care, 8
and new paradigm, 5–6
search for meaning, 5
three domains in, 35
self-help programs
and personal accountability, 12
and self-improvement programs, 12
spirituality in, 11–13
shamanism
and altered states of consciousness, 22
compared to modern health care, 23

shamanism *(continued)*
   in nursing history, 21–24
   realms of reality in, 22
   and spirits, 22–23
   trance state in, 22–24
soul
   Earth as learning environment for, 43
   in nursing theory, 115–116
spirituality
   and the brain, 79–91
   and care delivery models, 13–17
   and death and dying, 93–94,
   definition of, 1
   in developmental theories, 51–66
   diseases due to spiritual emergence,
      76–77
   and ethics, 185–192
   and healing, 129–137
   and history of nursing, 8–11, 21–33
   and holism, 89–91
   and illness, 93–96
   and managed care, 17
   and medical outcomes, 7
   and the mind, 71–77
   New Age elements, 7
   and Nightingale, 29–32
   and philosophy, 39–45
   and physics, 37–39
   and physiological correlates, 86–87,
      89–91
   and psychology, 45–47
   and psychotherapy, 73–75
   reality of spiritual experience, 86–87
   and reductionism, 87–89, 91
   renewed interest in, 5
   in self-help programs, 11–13
   *See also* new care delivery models,
      nursing history, nursing theories
spiritual theories, 10–11
spiritual therapeutics
   being and doing, 149–150
   bioenergetics, 151–156
   body-mind-spirit interface, 141–142
   giving meaning to illness and
      suffering, 170–171
   guided imagery, 147–149

helping the patient maintain faith,
   172
hypnotic regression, 145
and levels of spiritual/religious
   development, 176–177
and matters of conscience, 173
and medical mystics, 157–158
meditation, 150–151
New Age, 141–159
New Age and religious compared,
   173–174
prayer, 165–166
presencing, 166–167
psychologically oriented therapies,
   143–145
psychoneuroimmunoendocrinology,
   146–147
and religion, 163–180
religious contemplation, 167–169
religious counselors, 173
repatterning, 144–145
ritual, 169–170
role of patient, 157
and spiritual diagnoses, 142
traditional spiritual therapies,
   163–180
*See also* healing
substance abuse, and search for spirit,
   11–12, 75

T
therapeutic touch, 153–156
trance state
   in Greek practices, 24–25
   in shamanism, 22–24
transcendence
   and the ego, 63
   in Maslow's model, 55–56
   and transpersonal developmental
      model, 61–62
transpersonal psychology, 44
   in developmental theories, 62–63
   in nursing theory, 114–115, 120

W
wicca movement, 29

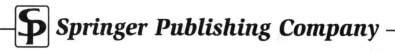 **Springer Publishing Company**

# Assessing and Measuring Caring in Nursing and Health Science

### Jean Watson, RN, PhD, HNC, FAAN

*"A magnificent job... Dr. Jean Watson and her colleagues have focused their careers on the phenomenon of caring, and this book is another one of their great contributions to the scientific community."*

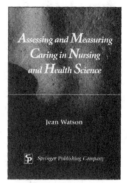

—From the Foreword by
**Ora L. Strickland,** RN, PhD, FAAN

Dr. Watson and colleagues have gathered all the available measurement instruments on caring in nursing in this book, where they are presented along with discussion of their origins, development, and use. Nurse clinicians, educators, researchers, and managers will find this a valuable resource.

**Partial Contents:**

**Part I: Overview**
- Caring and Nuring Science: Contemporary Discourse
- Background for Selection of Caring Instruments

**Part II: Summary of Each Instrument for Measuring Caring**

**Part III: Challenges and Future Directions**
- The Evolution of Measuring Caring: Moving Toward Construct Validity
- Postscript—Free Thoughts on Caring Theories and Instruments for Measuring Caring
- Appendix: Master Matrix Blueprint for All Instruments for Measuring Caring

Nurse's Book Selection • AJN Award Winner
2001   336pp   0-8261-2313-9   hard

11 West 42nd Street, NY, NY 10036 • www.springerpub.com
Order Toll-Free: 877-687-7476
Fax: (212) 941-7842  •  Tel: (212) 431-4370

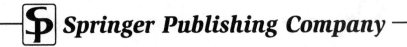
# Springer Publishing Company

# Encyclopedia of Complementary Health Practice

**Carolyn Chambers Clark,** EdD, RN, ARNP, FAAN, Editor in Chief
**Rena J. Gordon,** PhD, Contributing Editor
**Barbara Harris,** RN, LMT, and
**Carl O. Helvie,** RN, DrPH, Advisory Contributing Editors

This comprehensive resource of key terms and concepts in complementary health care addresses–practices, conditions, and research-based treatments. With over 300 entries by distinguished contributors, coverage includes such alternative therapies as naturopathy, homeopathy, chiropractic, nutrition, and massage.

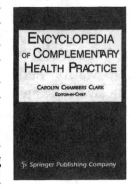

One section is devoted to pertinent issues in complementary health practice, including economics, legal ramification, education, and historical perspectives. Other valuable features are the extensive cross references and a directory of practitioners and institutes relevant to complementary health practice.

**Major Sections:**

**PART I: CONCEPTS AND ISSUES**
**PART II: CONDITIONS**
**PART III: INFLUENTIAL SUBSTANCES**
**PART IV: PRACTICES AND TREATMENTS**
**PART V: CONTRIBUTOR DIRECTORY**
**PART VI: RESOURCE DIRECTORY**

1999   664pp   0-8261-1239-0   soft   •   0-8261-1237-0   hard

11 West 42nd Street, NY, NY 10036 • www.springerpub.com
Order Toll-Free: 877-687-7476
Fax: (212) 941-7842 • Tel: (212) 431-4370